"Peter Barton and Laurence Shames, the graceful writer he persuaded to help him tell this tale, have produced a worthy monument, a book about how to live, and how to die." —Ken Auletta

"This is a wise, funny, and intensely true book—a generous gift from an amazing guy to those of us who are so busy getting through life that we sometimes forget why we're living. Sooner or later, we'll all make the journey Peter Barton took; now, thanks to him, it doesn't look so scary." —Dave Barry

"A little masterpiece. . . . A book to be read by everyone. . . . [It] may be the most honest book I have ever read. . . . Some of [the] phrases and sentences literally took my breath away. . . . [*Not Fade Away*] lit up my own mind and spirit—dare I include soul?—to consider my own life and purposes." —Jim Lehrer

"You couldn't know Peter Barton and not know he would face dying in the most adventurous and original way. . . . This is a book full of insight and comfort, wisdom and hope." —Barry Diller

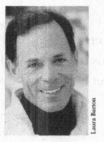
Laura Barton

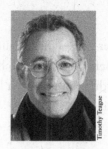
Timothy Teague

About the Authors

PETER BARTON (left) was a founder and CEO of Liberty Media and a passionate advocate for such innovative programming as the Discovery Channel, Fox Sports Net, Black Entertainment Television, and QVC. After leaving Liberty in 1997, he devoted himself to philanthropy and education. He taught a graduate business course in entrepreneurship at the University of Denver and founded the nonprofit Privacy Foundation. He died in September 2002.

LAURENCE SHAMES (right), formerly the Ethics columnist for *Esquire*, is a critically acclaimed novelist and essayist, and was the ghostwriter of the *New York Times* bestseller *Boss of Bosses*. He lives in Ojai, California.

NOT FADE AWAY

a short life

well lived

LAURENCE SHAMES

and

PETER BARTON

Perennial
An Imprint of HarperCollinsPublishers

FIRST PERENNIAL EDITION PUBLISHED 2004.

Designed by Leanne Coppola/Abbate Design

Library of Congress Cataloging-in-Publication Data

Shames, Laurence.
   Not fade away : a short life well lived / Laurence Shames and Peter Barton.— 1st Perennial ed.
          p. cm.
     ISBN 0-06-073731-X
     1. Barton, Peter, 1951–2002—Health. 2.
Stomach—Cancer—Patients—Colorado—Biography. I. Barton, Peter, 1951–2002. II. Title.9+

RC280.S8B377 2004
362.19699'433'0092—dc22
[B]

                                                                    2004044655

     15 16 17 18 ❖/RRD 12 11 10

To Laura, my absolute best friend, lover, partner, and wife.
And to Kate, Jeff, and Chris. You three are our proudest legacy
and greatest accomplishment.

—*P.B.*

To Marilyn, with love, as always. But even more so now.

—*L.S.*

Genevieve,

Words inside I know
you will appreciate.

~ Adriel

LIVE AS THOUGH YOU'LL LIVE FOREVER.
AND BE PREPARED TO DIE TOMORROW.

—*The Talmud*

LOVE IS LOVE AND NOT FADE AWAY.

—*Buddy Holly*

PREFACE

I TRIED MY DAMNEDEST NOT TO GET INVOLVED in the writing of this book, or with a man named Peter Barton, whose life it celebrates and whose death it chronicles.

My reason for resisting was simple: My own small existence was on a very pleasant, even keel; I didn't want to disrupt it by getting close to a dying stranger. I didn't want to think about mortality, still less watch death happening from day to day. I didn't want to grow to care about a family that would soon be fatherless.

Besides, I had no special reason to embrace Peter Barton's story. As of January 2002, when a mutual friend told me his disease was terminal, all I knew of Peter was that he was a media business mogul who lived in Denver. True, he seemed like an audacious and amusing character—a fellow whose edge had not been blunted by success, who'd preserved his healthy mistrust of authority, his almost boyish need to push the rules and test the limits. There were endless anecdotes about Peter: Peter rock-climbing up Robert Redford's chimney; Peter driving race cars, or flying off of ski jumps in his underwear; Peter winning a Rolls-Royce on a bet, or hatching wild but visionary schemes like buying public television to rescue it from spending cuts. . . .

Audacious, for sure. Amusing, yes, but what did it have to do with me? Peter's world was not my world; Peter's alpha-male style was not my style. We'd made vastly different choices in life. Peter built enterprises, wielded power; I worked alone and wanted control over nothing but myself. Peter, through his work and his children, had projected himself into the future; I had consciously abstained from fatherhood, and accepted with relief the idea that my stake in earthly matters would end the moment I did.

Even the things that Peter and I did have in common tended to make me shy of him—spooked me, in fact. It turned out we were almost exactly the same age, born a few months apart in the baby boom year of 1951. But Peter was already wasting away with stomach cancer. If it could happen to him—if Death was beginning to pluck at our still-youthful generation—

then why not me? Peter's skin was smoother than mine. He had less gray hair than I did.

So I had plenty of reasons to run from this story.

And yet I didn't run. Deeply if briefly—Peter was gone within seven months of the first time we ever met—I became immersed in his amazing life and courageously examined death. Why? Because I found that I could not do otherwise.

The main reason for this was Peter himself. The man was utterly compelling. He was brilliant; he was brash; he'd lived his life with pagan zest, and, even at the nadir of his sickness, he was incapable of feeling sorry for himself. As he grew more ill, he also grew more open. There was nothing, however intimate or painful, that Peter wouldn't talk about; there was no question that was disallowed.

Summing up his life, pondering what was to come, his moods and emotions all seemed outsized. He had a wicked temper, and a smile that lit the room. He was cocky and he was insecure, he was proud and he was modest. He could be wiltingly sarcastic and unashamedly affectionate, and his love for his family was almost frighteningly intense.

But the thing that won me over, finally, was that Peter, who'd grown up barely middle class and had had to scrap for everything he'd gained, had never stopped being one of us. For all his accomplishments, he was mainly just a guy you'd like to have a beer with, swap some jokes. I came to think of him as a sort of overachieving Everyman.

Nothing Peter did was ordinary, yet the hopes and needs that spurred him on were universal. If his triumphs were extreme, his dreams were touchingly typical. Zelig-like, he invented himself again and again, entered each new stage of life with a persona that seemed to suit it perfectly, and thus participated in his times more wholeheartedly than most of us dared.

Which of us garage musicians didn't dream of playing with a band that went on to be famous? Peter did that. Who among us hasn't entertained the fantasy of chucking everything, escaping to the Rockies, bumming around Aspen or skiing avalanche patrol in Idaho? Peter did that, too. Likewise, waiting till past thirty to choose a career. And conquering the business world with a sort of karmic wild-man irreverence—which is to say, by being entirely himself. And retiring at forty-six, with plenty of dough and a household full of love.

Thinking about the extraordinary degree to which Peter's life fulfilled the drives and ambitions of so many of us, I began to feel that his story was bigger than himself. It was also an accounting of the stunningly generous options available to a lucky generation—a sort of boomer fable. Hungry for experience, avid for life, Peter showed us what was possible.

But now he was dying. At fifty.

This huge, rude fact was appalling, inconceivable, wrong. Death was for old people, not for us. Death was for faded aunts and palsied uncles, for the parents we worry about so much.

Peter's dying at my age was a terrible mistake that made me want to mutter something sympathetic, and then go run and hide.

But again, I didn't hide. I couldn't hide. I drew ever closer to this dying man who had now become my friend, and I came to understand that he was offering me a difficult but extraordinary privilege: the chance to bear witness to an incomparable adventure, to observe—inasmuch as an outsider ever can—the progress of a journey that each of us will make, finally, alone.

Some people are born to lead and destined to teach. Peter Barton, I think, was one of these. He would have preferred, God knows, a longer life; but when he knew that he was dying—dying in the vanguard of his generation—he seemed to feel a responsibility to make his death of use. He set himself a final goal: to die well, with gratitude rather than complaint, with dignity and grace, with a highly personal faith that could coexist with reason. Though he never put it in these words, it seemed important to him to set a good example, to make of his passing a quiet lesson.

This book is the record of things Peter and I talked about and felt together in the last months of his life. During that time, and despite his waning strength, Peter lived with an amazing richness and intensity; life, for him, seemed heightened by the nearness of its end. He had no time for trivialities; his mind was fixed on large and final things. He spoke of love, family, value, spirit. He faced down fear at every moment, quested after peace with every breath. And, with an effort that seemed to me heroic, he battled horrific pain to preserve his clarity, so that he might send back honest dispatches from the frontier he was approaching.

Peter made me look at things I didn't know I had the nerve to look at. His rollicking, high-stakes life cast a strangely reassuring light on the smaller, quieter choices I had made. Studying the courage and the undaunted curiosity with which he moved toward death, I grew at least a little less afraid of my own mortality.

I failed, then, to resist this story. But I hope I've succeeded, at least, in being its faithful steward, in presenting it simply and candidly, as Peter wanted it to be. That's the least I could do for a man from whom I learned so much.

—L.S.

INTRODUCTION

M Y NAME IS PETER BARTON, and probably the first thing I should say is that I consider myself an incredibly lucky man.

I've got a wonderful wife and three great kids. I've done everything I ever wanted to do in life, and packed it into fifty-one years. There's not one thing I regret or wish I could redo. There's not one thing I wish I'd done, and didn't. I'm contented and fulfilled.

Not that life has come easily for me.

Some people are born vastly talented or congenitally confident. Not me. I was born with middling smarts; an unexcep-

tional degree of musical ability; a modest knack for sports. Whatever I did, I gritted out. I valued nonchalance, and I tried not to
let the effort show, but the fact is that I worked my butt off.
Faked confidence when I didn't really feel it. Contended at every
stage with my own insecurities and fear of failure.

I wouldn't—and couldn't—have had it any other way.
This is who I am, and it's way too late to start apologizing. I've
always been a striver who sometimes tried too hard, was at moments too feisty and too stubborn for my own good. I'm still
stubborn, frankly. Stubbornness is one of the things that keeps
my life feeling like my own.

As I say, though, I've been lucky, and that luck began on
the day I was born—because that day was right in the heart of
the baby boom. Let me say this straight out, because it's the big
context in which my own life has been just a tiny part: Our generation is the luckiest that ever lived. Way luckier than we did
anything to deserve.

We were born into a time of prosperity and peace. The
world seemed safe and was ours to explore. No one talked about
limits and boundaries. No one ever used the word *impossible*.
We were encouraged to pursue our dreams, in a world that only
got better.

We had amazing music, and free love that wouldn't kill
you. During the biggest crisis of our adolescence—Vietnam—we
linked arms and helped stop an ugly and immoral war. We

brought the races closer together, and gay people out of the closet. We had the blessing of living more openly and honestly than any generation that had gone before.

Perhaps the luckiest part of all was that we were the generation that wasn't rushed and bullied into becoming grown-ups too soon. We could knock around without guilt or undue anxiety. We could take the time—in the parlance of the day—to *find ourselves*. That phrase, I realize, has become one of ridicule, a way of deriding the navel-gazing of the sixties and seventies. But maybe it's time to reexamine that. What's unworthy about working to understand who you truly are and what you really want from life? What better use can a person make of his youth?

Anyway, we had the luxury of believing that, eventually, there would be a career, a track—but in the meantime there were a lot of excellent detours. I took my share of them, from the slightly crazy to the somewhat reckless, and sucked the marrow out of every one.

But while I was busily goofing off, something mysterious and amazing was happening—something I didn't even realize at the time. Gradually, on my own schedule and no one else's, I was becoming *ready*. Ready to be a responsible adult. Ready to be a husband. Ready to be a father. Ready to *work*—and to do so not in the drab spirit of trading time for money, but with the joyful ambition of creating something, participating in an enterprise I could be proud of.

On that front, things went better than I would have dared to hope. I helped to build, from almost nothing, a multibillion-dollar company called Liberty Media.

Unless you work in television or on Wall Street, it's possible you've never heard of Liberty. But if you've ever watched the Discovery Channel, or the Learning Channel, or MacNeil/Lehrer, or Fox Sports, or Home Shopping Network, or STARZ!, or Black Entertainment Television, you know some of what Liberty does. It's a powerful outfit that's done a lot to shape the media landscape, and I take enormous satisfaction from having been a part of it.

At the same time, while I was in business I always felt a little like a double agent. I wore a suit and tie but my spirit hopped around in a loincloth. A reconstructed hippie, I was doing this for the thrill of the game. As a deal maker, I could play at being a hard-ass when I had to, but I like to think I was at least a hard-ass with a notion of karma, a sense of fairness.

I was playing out the baby boomer dream of having it all ways, and by the time I left Liberty, at the age of forty-six, I felt like I'd already led two lives. One had been funky, the other was elegant, and I'd totally savored them both.

All in all, then, an amazing run of good fortune. But no streak lasts forever. There's always a bad break eventually.

For me, the bad break was cancer.

I've had it for more than three years now. We've had a seesaw battle, my disease and I. At times I really thought I was winning, really thought I'd *won*. Then the cancer would come back. There'd be another surgery, radiation, a regimen of chemo. The treatments weakened me as much as they theoretically hammered the disease. I never lost my will to fight, but I could feel my body gradually losing its ability to rally, to recover from each new assault.

Over time, I became strangely detached from my physical self. I came to feel like a passenger on a doomed airplane. Sitting there strapped into my seat, I've watched the engines flame out one by one. There's been nothing more that I could do.

In recent months the disease has progressed dramatically, kicked into a whole different gear, and now I seem to be dying.

I say "seem" because, while for the most part I accept the situation, there still are moments when I simply don't believe it. Some people might say that at such times I am "in denial." Well, "denial" is an easy word to use when it's not your own life hanging in the balance. I prefer to think that I am facing facts while waiting for a miracle.

That's right—a miracle.

Until quite recently, that word was not in my vocabulary. Truthfully, I'm uneasy with it even now. I'm a practical person, a skeptical person. I respect logic. I weigh odds. I examine facts and draw conclusions. I don't make wild leaps of reasoning, or faith.

Like so many of my peers, I've never wanted anything to do with organized religion. Too much hypocrisy; too much intolerance, way too many people killing and maiming in the name of God.

Equally, though, I've had a tough time warming up to contemporary spirituality. Too much psychobabble; too many buffoons pretending to be gurus. About the closest I've come to "religion" is a private ritual I've practiced these last fifteen years or so: I wish on stars, a different one each night.

Lately, though, I seem to be mellowing, opening myself to a wider range of possibilities.

It's not that I *believe*, exactly. But I've come to feel that nothing which gives comfort should ever be despised. Peace is to be cherished, however it's delivered. God, angels, forest sprites— bring 'em on! These days, I knock wood, I mumble litanies of the names of loved ones, old friends—this, for me, is praying.

People who've known me for a long time might think I'm going soft in the head. I prefer to see it as going tender in the heart.

My disease has been good for me in a certain sense. It has made me more accepting, gentler. Earlier in my life I might have been ashamed of this, seen it as a sign of weakness. Now I'm proud of it. It means I'm growing unafraid.

Unafraid to admit there are things I can't explain and will never understand. Unafraid to acknowledge that I can no longer control my destiny with street smarts and good thinking. Unafraid of the unknown place I'm moving toward.

—June 2002

NOT FADE AWAY

THE MAGIC'S IN THE MUSIC,
                    AND THE MUSIC'S IN ME . . .
                                                    —John Sebastian

♦♦♦

UNTIL I STARTED SPENDING TIME with Peter Barton, I'd never heard a dying man play rock 'n' roll.

But now, on a snowy winter afternoon in Denver, he struggled up from the couch where we'd been chatting, and in answer to some impulse he never bothered to explain, he went to the piano. He shook himself to gain some slack in the IV tubes running up his shrunken arms, and launched into a happy, raucous set.

Fittingly, he began with the Joe Cocker classic, "Feelin' Alright (Not Feelin' Too Good Myself)." Then he flung himself into an improvised medley that gathered up the music of a lifetime—the Beatles, Dave Brubeck, Motown, Frank Sinatra—and embraced each tune as if hugging an old friend.

He should not have been able to do this. His abdomen was clogged with cancer. He could no longer eat, and even with the intravenous feeding, he lost weight every day. The doctors no longer knew what to tell him, except that he was in the last months, possibly the last weeks, of his life.

Yet his playing was clean, assured, and *loud*, and its effect was utterly startling—as if the Last Trumpet had sounded, and a soul, joyously reunited with its long-discarded flesh, had roused itself and begun to dance.

It was when I heard Peter play the piano—listened to him beat back mortality, chord by chord—that I began to think of him as not just an interesting person but an extraordinary one. Another thought occurred to me as well: I wondered if perhaps everyone, facing death, became extraordinary; if maybe each of us had untapped reserves of nerve and strength that might prove surprising, even glorious, at the end.

His hands bony, his skin oddly translucent, Peter leaned into the Yamaha grand that shared his living room with assorted dog toys and children's playthings. Once he started playing it seemed like he could improvise for hours. It seemed, too, that he just didn't want to stop. I thought I heard a certain dread of stopping creep into the tunes, making them both more urgent and more solemn.

Seamlessly, he segued from Aretha Franklin to the Beach Boys, from Otis Redding to the Rascals. And I realized something very basic and very powerful: We knew all the same songs.

For all the differences in our chosen lives, we'd hummed the same tunes as we lived them. The same lyrics had first given words to my youthful longing and his; likewise to our discovery of lust, and frustration, and pain. Through the music, we knew a lot about each other before we'd said a word.

I stood there next to the piano, and at some point I could no longer help myself—I was playing air guitar and singing along. Peter threw his head back on his stringy neck and harmonized. To me, this was huge. Singing harmony with someone, inhabiting a chord together, is a perfectly intimate thing.

That day, and in the weeks that followed, Peter and I evolved a growing trust, a luxurious confidence that the other person got it, that let us speak a kind of shorthand. He talked about his childhood; he didn't need to say a lot, because his childhood was also mine, with its overriding tone of optimism and safety. He spoke of early hurts, humiliations—those painful episodes that everyone has and no one ever forgets. He reviewed the bewildering watershed moment when a child first learns that there is such a thing as loss.

He spoke of another sort of "childhood," as well—the infancy of his disease, and the surreal day he first learned of it.

Peter made me understand that, just as every life begins at a particular moment, so does every death. There is a heartbeat when the process starts, when a person makes the first dreaded stumble from health to sickness. An array of consequences fans out from that moment—physical, practical, emotional. Everything comes due for reconsideration. Time itself de-forms. The process is as complicated as life itself; it becomes, in fact, a sort of second life, running parallel to the life that one has lived so far. . . .

On that winter afternoon, however, Peter wasn't analyzing, wasn't talking much at all. He'd all but vanished into his beautiful, improbable music. Eyes closed now, he stitched "Take Five" onto "Midnight Hour," glided from "Desperado" to "Let It Be."

In one of our very first talks, a phone conversation before we'd ever met, Peter had told me almost defiantly that he was not a spiritual person and never had been. Listening to him play, I took the silent liberty of not believing him.

The music insisted otherwise. What is spirituality if not an ultimate willingness to reach deep? Peter at the keyboard was reaching deeper than anyone I'd ever seen—reaching straight past illness, past debility and death to joy and peace.

He played a final, mighty chord, then let his hands rest on the keys. He was slightly winded; his skin had a feverish gleam; I saw the pulse move in his neck. Behind him, through the west windows, the snowcapped Rockies were backlit by a wan and fading sun.

Peter shot me a smile I can only describe as otherworldly. "Man," he said, "where did that come from?"

1

You CAN TELL A LOT about a person by his nick-name, right?

Mine's Hawk. I've had that moniker for as long as I can remember, and it still tickles me. I just love the word. It conjures images of soaring flight against a cloudless sky. It implies a majestic independence, a raptor's uncompromising realism. . . .

Except that's not the kind of hawk I'm named after.

I'm named after the Studebaker Hawk, a market flop of a sport coupe that was manufactured in the middle 1950s. I just loved the name of the thing. It seemed to summarize all that was cool and jaunty.

Besides, it's really more fitting that I was named after a car. As a kid, I didn't soar, I rode around. I fantasized about automobiles, but what I rode was bicycles or motorized dinghies that I cobbled together from spare parts. Mine was a down-to-earth, nuts and bolts, tinkering kind of childhood.

Then again, kids are always soaring. For them, there's no boundary between the down-to-earth and the heavenly. Mud is a miracle. Snow is pure chilled joy. A pile of leaves is a sacred altar. Why do we lose that feeling, that sense of wonder, for so much of our lives?

Anyway, I was born in Washington, D.C., but while I was still an infant the family moved to Painted Post, New York, a tiny upstate town complete with maple trees and dappled cows and a beautiful white steeple. And pregnant women! Pregnant women carrying toddlers; pregnant women pushing strollers. There were a million kids to play with. Nice kids, nasty kids, gentle kids, bullies—all of human nature was represented in our little neighborhood.

Our family, in almost every way, was typical. My mother, in those years, was a housewife. My father worked too hard and wasn't around as much as I'd have liked. We were neither rich nor poor; I don't think I knew those categories existed. Everyone was middle class. Life got better for everyone together. One year there was television, the next year there was color television. One year Dad drove a shiny new Dodge, the next year there was a DeSoto with even bigger tail fins.

Kids don't know from economics, but here's the lesson I absorbed: Money needed to be worked for *but not fretted over*. It would appear when required. In the meantime, better to climb trees and build snowmen. In other words, to live.

But I want to tell you about Painted Post's one claim to fame. It is very near the Corning Glass factory, where my father worked.

In case there's anyone who doesn't remember, Corning did not begin with the fiber optics business. In the 1950s, Corning manufactured plates and platters and Pyrex pans. What the company was best known for, though, was casserole dishes. Everybody had them, remember? Their trademark was an abstract blue flower.

Since my dad worked for Corning, my mom had every casserole shape ever made. We had one for stew. We had one for soup. We had one for potatoes. If they'd made one for individual spaghetti strands, we'd have had that one too! I can still see the metal cradles that the dishes sat in at the table . . .

But wait—why am I going on about casseroles? I think it's because the approach of death has made me realize that there are no unimportant details in life. That childhood sense of wonder is somehow coming back to me. How can I put it?

Things, and the meanings that they have, are being reunited in my heart.

Those old casseroles—maybe they're just chipped and battered pans, but for me they're connected with incredibly precious things, giant notions like Mother, Kitchen, Family Meals.

So cut me some slack if I get nostalgic now and then over trivialities. The thing is, they don't seem trivial to me. I've come to feel that the big things in life are best understood by way of small things. Ignore the small ones, and the big ones just seem like fancy words, slogans without the truth of something you really know, and really feel.

◆ ◆ ◆

WHO KNOWS HOW OR WHEN a disease is actually born?

Who knows what cancer is like in its appalling infancy, when the first disastrous cell divisions are just starting to occur, before detection is possible?

For all I know, there may be something beautiful in the process. Under a microscope, in time-lapse, it might look like flowers opening, mushrooms burgeoning. Maybe that sounds creepy—but just because something's bad for us, that doesn't mean it can't be beautiful on its own terms. Nature is full of gorgeous and deadly things.

Whatever my disease's early history was like, here's how I first learned of it: My doctor called me on my cell phone.

It is Pearl Harbor Day, December 7, 1998. I'm forty-seven, and I've been supposedly "retired" for a year and a half. But I'm as busy as I've ever been. I've started foundations. I've been teaching a seminar in business school. I sit on boards of various corporations and advise many friends who are still in mid-career. I feel a joyful obligation to help out where I can. And, to tell the truth, I still love the action.

Today I'm in Silicon Valley, at an informal board meeting at Yahoo. They've asked me to become a director. This is flattering, but I pass—mainly because their business model scares me. How can they actually make money? That's what we're talking about on this particular afternoon: formulating an economic model for a big aggregation of e-commerce businesses. This excites me. What I like is creating things, adding value, shaping the big picture. I'm there to brainstorm, to enjoy the company of some really smart people. And to suggest to them some big ideas—which, I conclude, they're not ready for.

What I have to say, basically, is that what Yahoo has done so far is just one piece of a puzzle. Everyone knows their name, but where do they exist, what do they *do*? I'm telling them they need to become a media company. They need broadcasting. They need content. They've got two choices: become marginal, or go head-to-head with AOL and Microsoft.

At some point the meeting becomes electric. This happens every now and then in business, and when it does, it's an adrenaline rush for sure. It happens when Big Stuff is on the table and people know that the brains and resources are there to do it, if only the will can be found . . .

And that's when my cell phone rings.

As a matter of policy, I turn my phone off when I go into a meeting. This one time I forgot. And at this crucial moment the damn thing starts buzzing away. I'm slapping at pockets, poking at buttons. I can't get it to stop. Finally I answer, just to make it shut up.

It's a doctor of mine in Denver. I barely know him. He barely knows me. I don't go to doctors very much. Why would I? I'm a healthy guy, a fitness nut. I'd gone to see him because I had a little bellyache.

"Mr. Barton?" he says.

"Speaking."

"I need you to come to my office to discuss this with me. You have cancer."

Just like that. That terse; that quick; that casual.

I don't remember getting up, but suddenly I'm standing. The Yahoo board of directors is staring at me. Maybe they understand that something bad has happened; maybe they're just wondering what could possibly be more important than going head-to-head with AOL.

I leave the meeting. I'm not dizzy, exactly, but out in the hallway the floor doesn't seem quite level, the walls meet the ceiling at a peculiar angle. I've still got the doctor on the phone, but he refuses to say much. It's my life, but we're doing this his way. He insists he needs to see me in his office.

I head for my plane. On the way, I feel my stomach, pat it down as if searching for a loaded weapon. Somewhere in there— somewhere in *me*—something poisonous is growing.

This is inconceivable and horribly insulting. It was just a little bellyache that lingered. No shooting pain, no fever. Nothing more than a vague feeling of wrongness in my gut.

It couldn't be cancer. It had to be some grotesque mistake.

2

W HEN DOES A CHILD first begin to understand that things change, that people and places come and go? For me, it happened on moving day.

I was five, in the middle of my kindergarten year. My family was moving to a modest house in Old Greenwich, Connecticut. I didn't understand why we had to go. I was told my father needed to be closer to Manhattan.

Moving men loaded up the furniture. My parents packed a million small things in the car, including me and my baby brother, John. When we pulled away from the house, I got a lump in my throat that took me totally by surprise, and returns even now as I think of it.

I was doing something I'd never done before: closing off a chapter of my life. Saying a real good-bye. Not *see ya later*. Good-bye.

Kindergarten friends—gone, never to be seen again. My favorite climbing tree—never to be climbed again. The view out my bedroom window—vanished as if it had never been.

It was my first hint that life takes back what it gives. A hard lesson, but a necessary one. Things we've loved get lost, or traded in. The stories of our lives have a due date, like books at the library.

But, anyway, people of happy temperament find ways to be happy, and I was basically a cheerful kid. Old Greenwich turned out to be just fine. To my amazement, I made new friends. There were different woods to walk through, and a salt pond where you could catch minnows with a worm, a string, and a paper clip.

I was a baseball nut. And a Yankees fan, of course. I knew every player, his number and position. First base, number 14, Moose Skowron. Behind the plate, Yogi Berra, number 8.

But my hero was Bobby Richardson, the second baseman, number 1. He was a little guy, baby-faced. Not a power hitter but a scrapper. All heart. A kid could only admire Mickey Mantle; he could *be* Bobby Richardson.

So of course I played second base in Little League.

And this, unfortunately, brings me to one of the most excruciating incidents of my childhood—one of those awful moments, totally trivial in itself, that you literally spend your whole life getting over. I tell this story as a plea to parents, coaches, teachers: For God's sake, be careful what you say when a child messes up!

Here's the scene: A miniature New England ballpark. The grass a little ratty; a few lumps in the infield. Several rows of aluminum bleachers back the chain-link dugouts. Summer dusk. The lights are coming on. Crickets start scraping; I tell myself it's the buzz of the crowd.

The "crowd," though, is maybe a dozen people. Parents. Among them is my father.

It's the only game all season he's been able to attend. He's tried to get to others, but things always came up—trains that ran late, unexpected meetings, all the mundane distractions that prevent fathers from seeing their kids grow up, that fill them with regret years later. Now he's here and I desperately want to show him something.

It's the sixth and final inning. At this level of baseball, most batters strike out, and I haven't had an infield chance all game. I've stood there in my Bobby Richardson stance and done absolutely zilch. Now there's one out. Two.

The next batter finally makes contact.

He hits a grounder that's headed straight toward me. There's really no such thing as a routine play in Little League, but this comes pretty close. The ball's rolling, not skipping; there's no tricky spin; it's an easy play. Except that it's the last out, and the guy who records the last out is automatically a hero. And my father's watching.

The ball seems to take a long time to get to me. I reach down my glove to snare it. Somehow I fail to squeeze the catch. The grounder escapes the pocket of my mitt and rides up toward my wrist. My composure gone in a heartbeat, I grope to capture the ball against my skinny chest.

I still have time to make the play, but now I'm panicked. I forget everything I know about the simple throw to first. I let fly an ugly, misdirected toss that sails over the first baseman's head. The runner cruises into second.

I stand there looking at the ground. That's it. I've failed. I had my chance to be the hero, to make my father proud, and I blew it.

But the worst part was what happened next. Our coach, one of those grown-ups who cared about winning a lot more than the kids did, yelled out to the pitcher, "Come on, Andy. Looks like you'll have to finish it yourself."

As if I didn't just screw up *one* time, I'd screw up every time. No confidence. No faith.

I heard it. My father heard it. Everybody heard it.

That happened forty-three years ago. Between then and now I've succeeded at a lot of things that matter more than Little League. But not only do I still recall that incident, I'm still humiliated by it. I think of that botched play and I still feel shame, in the form of a tingling sensation at the back of my neck. Crazy, maybe, but there it is. That's how tender kids are.

◆◆◆

WE ALL KNOW, I guess, how easily wounded a child is; yet probably all of us, even with the best intentions in the world, cause our children pain. Or rather, life hurts them in the same ways it wounded us, but now it is us, the parents, who are the vehicles of life's hard messages.

Almost from the first moment I learn that I have cancer, my wife, Laura, and I are haunted by this question: How will we tell the children?

How can we be honest with them without scaring them into nightmares? How can we prepare them for what might happen, without making them sadder than we can bear to see? In December 1998, our daughter, Kate, is eleven. Our boys, Jeff and Chris, are nine and almost seven. How much can they understand? How much do they need to know?

We live with these questions for more than a year. In some ways, I think, it's a much harder year for Laura than for me.

All I have to worry about is the possibility of dying. She has to think about the far more complicated task of carrying on, taking care of everyone. Being a mother to children who could soon be fatherless. Being caretaker of a sick man who could get a great deal sicker. Facing the prospect of becoming a widow in the most vibrant time of her womanhood.

I tell myself that maybe we'll both be spared those terrible adjustments, those dreadful conversations. Because I firmly believe I have a damn good chance of beating the disease.

My hope is that someday, in the safety of past tense, we'll tell our children, *Dad had cancer, but now he's fine.*

And I'll tell my wife, *It's okay, now. I'll stay with you forever.*

In the meantime, though, I am living in doctor hell.

There is a feeling in this country that only the wealthy get top-notch medical care. Let me correct that impression. *No one* gets top-notch care—unless he fights hard for it at every juncture, and educates himself. The good news is that you need to become an expert only in the disease you have.

My gastroenterologist sends me to the surgeon he prefers. The surgeon tells me approximately where my tumor is. I ask him how he intends to treat it. He takes out a sheet of paper and draws a rough sketch of the human G.I. tract. As he's doing so—I am not making this up!—I notice a distinct tremor in his right hand. The guy can hardly hold a pencil and he's going to take a scalpel to my belly?

He indicates the place where the esophagus joins the stomach. "This is the gastroesophageal junction," he says.

He points to where the stomach is linked to the intestines. "And this is the pyloric valve."

Now he points to both valves at once. "I make a little snip *here*, and a little snip *here*, and then I resection what's left."

"You remove my entire stomach?"

"Yes, I think that's best."

"Doc, if you don't mind my asking, how many of these have you done?"

"Two or three," he says.

"I'll get back to you. If the phone doesn't ring, it's me."

I start doing research on the Internet. I call a few close friends. One, a cancer survivor himself, informs me that I'm going to Sloan-Kettering and nowhere else. He calls his own surgeon as if summoning the Messiah. This is the doctor-on-a-pedestal thing, big time. If it isn't voodoo, it's pretty close. Belief in the cure is part of the cure.

So I go to New York. And the operation, in fact, is a great success. The tumor is gone, and I'm left with at least some part of my stomach. No radiation or chemo is required at this point. If the cancer doesn't return within twelve months, there's a 90 percent chance I'll be okay. If I'm clean after three years, I won't even need further checkups.

Great news. But there's a recovery period from abdominal surgery, and I need a cover story. I'm not ready to be outed as a cancer patient—and for a very good reason.

One of the insidious things about cancer is that, even as it's leeching onto your body, it's subsuming your identity as well. In the eyes of others, you become the disease. People look at you and see cancer. That's all they want to talk about, as if you've already left the wider world behind, as if you're no longer a part of any other subject.

So my wife and I decide that, since I seem to be cured, we'll tell the kids I had an ulcer.

I say the same thing to associates. I make a joke of it. *I thought I was the guy who gave ulcers. Now I've got one.* It's a weak joke, but at least it ends discussions; it spares everyone the discomfort that goes with confronting serious illness.

I heal up well from the surgery—I'm still a young, healthy guy, right?—and soon I'm once again running myself ragged with my kids. Playing football, taking ski vacations, coaching my daughter's lacrosse team. I've always cherished family time, but now it's even sweeter.

Yet all the while that question simmers: What'll it be like if the cancer returns and we really have to prepare Kate and Jeff and Chris?

More than anything, I dread the thought that someday my children might look at me and see not their father but an illness; not the doting dad ready to throw a ball or nag them about their homework, but only the humiliated, emaciated, undignified walking corpse that a cancer victim eventually becomes.

3

PASSIONS TEND TO COME and go in life. Hobbies grab you for a while and then lose their fascination. Thank God, though, there are certain pleasures that never seem to fade, whose excitement lasts as long as life itself.

For me, the clearest case of this is music. I've loved it ever since I was a little kid; I love it just as much today.

Some years ago, I built myself a little barn—a combination art studio, workshop, and office—about a hundred yards from my house. I put in a set of kick-ass speakers, and I still sneak out there when I want to crank up some rock 'n' roll. It's sort of funny—I'm the dad now, my life is pretty close to over, but I'm still exiled to my room when I want to blast my music. Otis Redding. The Rolling Stones. My kids can't stand what I listen to.

Which is typical, right? That's proof of music's amazing power. It's part of how each generation defines itself. Every good song ever written is a kind of anthem of independence.

Music was both a bond and a huge issue between my father and me. Now that I think of it, everything that a son goes through with his father—wanting to please him, needing to break away; trying to be good enough, needing to be bad enough—was played out through the music.

My father was an incredible pianist, just a notch below concert grade. He'd been classically trained in Europe. He had perfect pitch. Now and then I'd walk past his study door and hear him chuckling. I'd peek in to find him reading a Beethoven or a Haydn score, laughing aloud like it was a Dave Barry column. He'd look up with an expression of pure heavenly pleasure on his face. "God," he'd say, "this is just so *witty*!"

So of course, starting at age seven, I was given piano lessons. And of course I hated them. Classical music was my father's thing; ergo, it couldn't be mine. My teacher was a conceited pedant who insisted on being called Doctor. Exercises were played by rote. Rhythm was dictated by the metronome. It was torture. What made it worse, of course, is that I knew I'd never be nearly as good as my father was.

In fairness, my lessons were probably as painful to my dad, with his perfect pitch, as to me. Practicing, I'd hit a wrong note and hear an anguished shout from some other part of the house: *That's a G! Play G!* This did nothing for my confidence.

Inevitably, I rebelled. At some point I refused to take any more lessons from the Doctor. My father, I'm sure, was crushed, but he came up with a Solomonic compromise: I could quit lessons as long as I didn't quit playing. I could play whatever music I liked, but the piano must remain a part of my life. On that my father was immovable.

I realize now something I didn't realize then: My father was determined to give me a gift. He was not generally affectionate; he wasn't lavish with his attention or his praise. This was his way of loving.

To him, music was the most sublime thing in the world; it was the most precious thing he could pass along. If I wouldn't accept the gift on his terms, he'd offer it on mine. If I threw it back in his face, he'd dust it off and present it again.

Like many kids, I was insufficiently grateful because I just didn't understand the value of what I was being given.

Gradually, though, I understood. I found a new piano teacher—a fabulous musician who was practically a bum, and was a perfect emblem of my musical rebellion. He smoked cheap cigars and stank of gin and my mother was reluctant to let him in the house. His clothes were threadbare and he never seemed to change them. He was so fat that his belly pressed against the keyboard, and his fingers were so thick that I was always surprised they didn't spread across two keys. But, man, could he play! He didn't care about proper fingering and he seldom bothered with written music. He improvised. He created. He taught me how to play the piano as intimately and personally as if I were singing.

And, ironically, he proved my father right about the life-long preciousness of music. Sometimes a seeming subversive turns out to be a parent's best ally.

Before I leave this subject of music and my father, there's one brief anecdote I want to tell. It's one of my most cherished memories. I didn't have a lot of perfect moments with my dad, but this was one of them.

It was 1964. I was thirteen. I'd just recently started playing with my first rock band; we called ourselves the Monarchs, which, at the time, we thought was pretty cool. But a piano wasn't very practical when you rehearsed in people's garages and played gigs at backyard barbecues. So, by default, I became the bass player.

Bass came pretty easily to me—it was just the left-hand piano part. The only problem was, I didn't own a bass. I borrowed gear from a rich kid who had a lot of instruments he couldn't play.

My father was away on one of his frequent business trips, a months-long one to the Far East. On the day of his return, my mom and I went to meet him at the airport.

He got off the plane with his briefcase in one hand and a guitar case in the other. I saw that case and my pulse started racing, I felt the excitement at the backs of my knees. It seemed like forever, watching him come down the ramp to approach us.

He gave us hugs then started chatting with my mother.

"Dad," I said, "what's in the case?"

"Case?" he said, like he had no idea what I was talking about. He went back to his conversation.

"The *guitar* case!" I said, pretty shrill by now.

"Oh. *That* case," he said.

And, very slowly, he went over to a row of plastic chairs in the waiting area and laid the guitar case across three seats. He snapped open the latches, one by one, then finally opened the lid. There, lined in flame-red plush, was a six-string Hoffner bass. A Hoffner! That's what Paul McCartney played! I mean, how cool was that?

For a moment I just stood there. I literally could not move. The bustle of the airport seemed to stall. The noise went silent. Finally I reached out and touched the bass, ran my fingers over the frets.

"Like it?" said my father.

I raised my eyes from the instrument and looked up at my dad. A couple of months is a long time in the life of a thirteen-year-old. Things change fast. In a way that I couldn't quite pin down, I felt that my father and I were looking at each other in a different way than before.

Thinking about it now, I realize that in giving me that bass he was saying, *It's okay, Pete. Be who you are.*

My father died a few months later. In the intervening years, I have bought, sold, smashed, and given away I don't know how many guitars. But I always kept that bass. It traveled with me; it stood in my study, still in its original red-plush case.

I finally gave it away this year. I gave it to my nephew Fred, who has a garage band of his own. My father's name was also Fred. It tickles me to pass along the gift of music to another generation.

◆ ◆ ◆

WHILE I'M TALKING ABOUT GIFTS, there's a side of having cancer that may sound fairly weird, but it's every bit as true as the fact that cancer is killing off my body: The experience of having this disease has done a lot of wonderful things for me, has led me to develop and grow in ways that might never have happened otherwise.

Somebody once quipped—and not at all facetiously—that there's one good thing about cancer: it doesn't kill you all at once. It gives you time to set your house in order—practically, emotionally, spiritually. It gives you time to think, to sum things up.

Socrates said that "the unexamined life is not worth living." Well, in the jam-packed decades before I got sick, my life went pretty unexamined. I was always moving fast, driving hard.

I didn't reflect; I was too busy *doing*. My energies went toward piling up experience, not toward finding meaning.

If I thought about meaning at all, I guess I imagined that someday it would just appear, that there would come a stage of life when the pieces of the puzzle would mysteriously resolve into something grander, something whole, something that, in a final way, *made sense*.

Except it doesn't happen like that.

I realize now that reflection is hard and active work. It calls for feats of memory and leaps of intuition. It takes imagination, and guesswork, and the humbling acceptance that there are things, even about oneself, that one will never understand.

Cancer is what brought me to that acceptance.

Let's for a moment go back to the end of 1998.

I've had my first big surgery. The docs tell me that my chances of a full recovery are very good. I can hardly describe the happiness I feel, the *lightness*. I feel not just reprieved, but reborn.

In ways subtle and otherwise, everything has changed.

Armed with my phony ulcer story, I go to cocktail parties. In the course of small talk, people tell me their problems—job stuff, investment stuff. I stand there with a serene and probably slightly smug smile on my face.

I'm thinking to myself: You think *that's* a problem? You're letting something like that make you unhappy? Buddy, you don't know what a problem *is*.

At the same time, I begin to notice certain things I'd never paid attention to before—because they hadn't applied to me. I come to understand that many people go through life just not feeling well. Chronic pain. Subtle and progressive maladies. Illnesses both physical and psychological that siphon off energy and strength.

I come to realize that, up until now, I've been guilty of the arrogance of health.

I've been impatient with people who didn't move as fast as I did, dismissive of people who couldn't do what I found easy. Now I understand that many of the things I took for granted are, for many people, monumental struggles. Simple things like climbing stairs, putting on clothes, even digesting food—for many people these acts require a kind of quiet heroism.

My compassion increases. I've always loved my family and my friends, but now I feel a warmth, even toward strangers, that wasn't there before.

Along with this, something even better happens. I feel an ever-increasing appreciation of human dignity. Forced to recognize that I, too, am fragile, I look more closely than I ever have at the troubles people go through—how patient they are in their suffering, how bravely they confront their burdens, how untiringly they support their loved ones. Everywhere I look, I see examples of courage and acceptance.

I am ever prouder to be human.

4

THERE'S AN OLD IRISH PROVERB: **He who is certain to**
die by flood needn't be afraid of fire.

I always knew my life would be a short one. But I never
gave a single thought to cancer. I was absolutely certain it would
be a heart attack that killed me.

My father died of a heart attack at forty-five. So had his
father before him. So, I thought, would I. This was destiny in the
form of genetics.

Understand, I didn't take this lying down. I did everything
I could to promote my cardiovascular health. I jogged, I rowed,

I spent endless hours on a bicycle. Cigarettes were anathema, of course. I deprived myself of butter and Brie, ate red meat only sparingly, kept my cholesterol levels in the best part of the range. The irony is that my ticker is so healthy that when the rest of me expires they'll probably have to beat it to death with a stick!

Looking back, it's clear to me that my father's death was one of the most pivotal events of my own life—maybe *the* most pivotal. It was my father's early passing that persuaded me to live as if my life was an extended two-minute drill with no time-outs, to cram a full span's worth of living into fifty years or even less.

Equally, though, my father's death brought my childhood to a cruelly sudden end.

For most kids, I think, childhood sort of tapers off; kids let go of it little by little, knowing that they're free to backslide now and then into silliness, into irresponsibility.

Which is how it *should* be. Adulthood is a big job; there should be a break-in period, an apprenticeship. But it didn't happen that way for me.

In a heartbeat I went from being a pretty carefree kid in a relatively secure environment to feeling totally responsible for my mother and two younger brothers. This was a hell of a thing for life to do to a kid, but there's no sense complaining about it. It's a big part of what made me who I am.

I remember the night my father died as though it happened yesterday.

I was staying over at a friend's house. At around three A.M. his parents woke me up and told me I had to go home. I had no idea why. I was groggy, disconnected. They bundled me into a car.

Before we reached my house, I saw the spinning lights on the tops of the police cars. They threw crazy, stretched-out shadows of shrubs and trees. We had to park across the street. I must have known that something awful had happened, because I could hardly get my legs to move.

A big cop was stationed on my porch. He stood above me and asked me who I was. I told him I was Peter. He sat down with me on the stoop and told me my father had died. He was a kind man and he said it as gently as he could. But there's no kind way to pass along a piece of news like that.

I couldn't process it; I went into a kind of stupor. Looking back, I think I stayed in that stupor for months, maybe even years.

I heard my mother crying upstairs. This was a sound I'd never heard before, and one I've never forgotten. I remember having the first, wildly confused thoughts about what I could do to comfort her. I was a little boy, after all. Should I put my arm around my mother? What could I possibly do to help?

The day of the funeral was probably the most baffling and overwhelming of my life.

I was dressed up, of course, and trying to be very brave. There were a lot of people at the funeral. Most of them I barely knew: business associates, people who claimed to be good family friends, though I never saw them again.

Before and after the ceremony, a procession of people came up to me. For the most part they were big, tall men who looked even more gigantic in their stuffed-shoulder suits. They squatted down to look me in the eye, put their huge hands on my skinny little shoulders, and all said pretty much the same thing: Son, you are now the man of the house. Take care of your mother and your brothers.

I suppose they meant well, but what a cruel and stupid thing to say to a little boy.

Enough grown-ups said that to me that I became convinced it was what I had to do. That's how the world worked. That's what was expected. Without a father, I was suddenly a man.

From that moment forward I felt like I had to take care of everything. If the stove didn't work, I had to figure out how to fix it. If my mother's car needed an oil change, I had to change the oil. I had to fix my brothers' bicycles, and if the younger kids got out of line, I had to go from being a co-conspirator to a disciplinarian. I had to put on a kind of adult solemnity, and half the time I couldn't tell if I was faking it or not.

And I learned how miserable it is, how life-draining, to worry about money.

My father's modest estate was poorly handled, and after he died I really thought we were going straight from Greenwich, Connecticut, to the poorhouse. My mother fretted over bills; at moments she seemed almost overwhelmed by her new responsibilities. At thirteen, I didn't see how I could help very much, other than by expanding my paper route. But I saw my mother worrying, and I worried alongside her.

I resolved then that someday, somehow, I would make enough dough so that everyone in my family would be provided for, that no one would have to worry the way we worried in those awful months.

That's the only part of having money that's ever mattered a damn to me.

♦♦♦

I'VE TRIED HARD not to blame my father for dying, not to be angry with him for leaving us.

Now the tables are turned. I'm the one abandoning my kids before a father should. More than anything, I hope my children won't think unkindly of me for that.

So I say this to Kate and Jeff and Chris: I've tried to be as present as I could for as long as I could. Forgive me that I couldn't be here longer. God knows that one of my very few regrets is that I won't be around to see more of your lives unfold.

At least I've had the opportunity to prepare my kids in a way that I was unprepared. Again, this is one of cancer's kindnesses. As my illness has progressed, so has my children's capacity to understand what's happening. Laura and I have had the luxury of time to decide what to say to them, and when. This story will not have a surprise ending, no numbingly sudden twists.

Not that I kid myself that anyone is ever totally ready for the death of a family member. Death, by its nature, is always abrupt. However gradual the process leading up to it, there comes a single moment when life ends. That moment can't be other than shocking. That's just how it is.

Still, I've had the luxury of being able to revisit what was most hurtful in my own father's passing, and to try, at least, to spare my family some of it. I have the enormous comfort of knowing that financial hardship won't be added to emotional pain, that I've seen to the practical matters a grieving family shouldn't have to worry about.

And I've had time to consider my good-byes, to say them not in a panicked, gasping rush, but little by little, in gestures and anecdotes, as things occur to me.

Here, for instance, as I think about my father and the things he didn't live to say, are some messages I want to make sure my kids and my wife hear loud and clear.

To my boys, I say this: Don't let anyone tell you that you've suddenly become little men, just because your dad is gone. You're still kids. Enjoy it. Goof off. Someday you'll realize you've become grown-ups, and you'll be proud of that. But let it happen on your own time, not anybody else's.

In the meantime, if something breaks around the house, you'll find a surprising satisfaction if you can fix it. But don't feel like you have to. There's no shame in calling the repairman!

To my daughter, I say this: When I first got sick you were a little girl. I've lived long enough to see you become a beautiful young woman. For this alone, I am eternally grateful to have had these last few years. I think it's okay with Mom if I say you are my best girlfriend and favorite date.

To my wife, I say this: If you feel like crying, please do it in a joyful, cleansing torrent and have it over with. Know that I am optimistic about what's happening, about where I'm going. It's an adventure, and I have always liked adventures.

I believe that there's Another Side. I wouldn't call it Heaven, and I'm not making any guesses about what it's really like. I'm pretty dubious about the harps and wings. I can take or leave the choir, unless it's gospel.

But I do believe that souls are reunited there.

So I'll wait for you at the end of the jetway. I'll chill champagne for the moment you rejoin me.

But there's no hurry. Love your life. Take your time.

It's funny in a way. In life, I've been the world's most in-a-hurry person. Death, I think, will teach me patience.

Better late than never.

CARPE DIEM. SEIZE THE DAY, BOYS!
MAKE YOUR LIVES EXTRAORDINARY.

—Tom Schulman, *Dead Poets Society*

◆ ◆ ◆

ONE DAY, AS OUR FRIENDSHIP was developing, Peter and I challenged each other—maybe even tested each other.

It was one of those times when men put their cards on the table, when the stylized exchanges of polite conversation fall away and what's left is a wonderfully incautious probing of what is really in another person's heart.

We were strolling the perimeter of Peter's property. It was a late winter day masquerading as spring. The air was warm, but an entire season's snow still blanketed the mountains. Underfoot, the grass was brown but springy with the miracle of returning life. Every breath smelled of promise as yet unfulfilled.

Peter walked slowly under the weight of a knapsack slung across his shoulder. The pack contained the pumps and tubes that were keeping him hydrated and somewhat nourished. But he hated the apparatus of his illness; he didn't want to inflict the sight of it on others; he tried his best to keep it tucked away.

Very considerate—but for myself, I found the knapsack heartbreaking. It made Peter look like a kid. He might have been heading for school with a bagful of books and an apple, or maybe playing hooky, sneaking off to the foothills for a hike among the earliest wildflowers and the gurgling rush of snowmelt streams.

I heard myself blurt out, "Peter, why are you doing this?"

He didn't answer right away. He was looking at a pair of

turtles that had trundled out of his pond and were sunning themselves on a log. Finally he said, "Hm?"

"This book," I said. "Spending time with me. There are lots
of other things you could be doing. Why is this important to you?"

He looked at me sideways and narrowed his eyes. A hint
of a sly smile crossed his face, and I had the distinct impression
I'd given him an opening he'd been waiting for. "I'll tell you," he
said. "But first I want your answer to the exact same question."

He stared at me a moment, then very patiently sat down
on a stump. I sat down next to him, hip to hip. There were, I suppose, a number of ways I might have answered. But I suddenly felt
it was time to tell Peter about the deaths of my mother and father.

A few years ago, in a horrific eight-month span, both my
parents passed away. Before that happened, I hadn't given much
thought to death. Like most people, I'd fended off such thoughts.
The topic was unpleasant, after all. And frightening. And besides,
I was too busy living, chasing this goal and that ambition, as if it
would go on forever.

Watching my parents die, I had no choice but to ponder
what was happening. Life did end. If my parents were dying, then
so would I someday. Elementary, sure, but how many people
truly grasp that simple fact before it's thrust into their faces?

In the aftermath of my parents' deaths, I was sadder than
I had ever been. I had aching dreams of impossible reunions. I
teared up listening to music. There were old black-and-white
photos I just couldn't bring myself to look at.

Gradually, though, the grief subsided—didn't go away, but was relieved of its harshness and became a warm smooth sense of loss, a kind of melancholy yet oddly welcome companion. And I discovered something that took me totally and utterly by surprise: The experience of seeing death up close had made my life better.

I found that I was calmer, less easily distressed by unessential things. My life grew both sparser and richer. There were fewer things I cared about, but those I valued seemed more precious than ever. I had a more vivid appreciation of health and time; among human virtues I now gave a higher rank to kindness.

And, at least to some degree, I was less controlled and driven by a fear I'd tried to keep a secret from myself.

There is nothing more humbling than an awareness of death. Death is the opponent that every single one of us will lose to. It's not a pretty fact, but once you get it through your head you begin to live more honestly.

Sitting on that log in warmth and sunshine that was far too stunning to last, Peter heard me out. He watched the turtles and squinted toward the gleaming mountains. His only answer was a small and thoughtful nod.

After a moment, I said, "Your turn."

He drew a deep and labored breath, let it out with a slight whistle, and hitched his shoulder to adjust the knapsack.

"I've got a few reasons for doing this," he said. "First, most important, I want my kids to know who their old man was. I want them to know something about my life, what I thought, what I valued. I want them to know how much I love them, how much I love their mother."

He broke off, looked away. His gaze seemed to fall on a young ash tree, the tips of its twigs just swelling into buds.

After a moment he continued. "And I want to get my two cents in about the amazing times we've been fortunate enough to live through. Not as an exercise in nostalgia, but for what it means now. Younger people today seem more passive, less hopeful than we were. That's a waste. I happen to believe that people can still choose the life they want. I wish I could persuade at least a few of them to get excited, get hyper, about their possibilities."

Peter, I mused, was the perfect pitchman for the benefits of being hyper. In our recent conversations he'd been revisiting his adolescence, the time when his hurry-up philosophy was born. Like most of us, he'd had more energy in those years than he well knew what to do with. You could only burn so much on rock 'n' roll. There was still plenty left to spend on bewilderment, and frustration, and the exhausting process of elbowing your way into your place in the world.

Peter's illness, too, had undergone a sort of "adolescence"—a period when too much was changing too fast, and the only possible reaction was an unproductive anger, a helpless rage that Peter had spoken about with disarming candor.

He discussed his turmoil as readily as his triumphs. He freely admitted when he'd been emotionally stymied, or when a lesson had been learned too late. He could be awfully hard on himself, utterly unsparing. Why? I came to understand that a little better as we continued our stroll around the pond on that unseasonable day.

"There's one more reason I'm doing this," said Peter. "Don't laugh. I'd really like to do something important before I die."

I didn't laugh, but I expect my eyes got wide. "You've already done a lot of important stuff."

"Have I?" he said. "The business stuff? The television stuff? Look, I'm proud of what I've accomplished. A lot of it was creative. I've made a lot of people financially secure. But was it important?"

It was Peter's question; only Peter could answer it. I just stood there looking at the mountains.

After a moment, he went on. "Look, I don't kid myself that my little death is any more important than those of the five or six billion people who've died before me. And I don't pretend to any special wisdom about what's happening. But that's the whole point, isn't it? I'm just one more person dying, trying to make sense of what I'm going through. The things I'm thinking, feeling—they're probably pretty typical of what anyone would think and feel.

"So if we just tell the story straight, without setting me up as some sort of guru, then I think there's something of value to be done, something that might be of help to others. Am I kidding myself?"

I put a hand on Peter's shoulder. "If you are," I said, "then at least there's two of us."

5

ADOLESCENCE, what a baffling time. Excruciating.

I sometimes think about those insects that are allowed to chill out in a nice, opaque cocoon between one stage of life and another. That's an extremely merciful provision of nature—from which we humans are unfortunately excluded. *We* have to go through our growing pains in plain sight of the world. And it isn't pretty.

Adolescence was when I first adopted my double-time approach to life. As I've said, this had nothing to do with a premonition of cancer, but with my father's heart attack. The Barton men just suddenly keeled over. If I was going to have my fair share of living, I'd have to pack twice as much experience into half as many years.

This was both a conscious stratagem and something far less manageable than a rational plan. The hurry-up philosophy allowed me to control my life, or to think I was controlling it; looking back, I was equally controlled by it. I put an awful lot of pressure on myself. Maybe that's partly why I eventually got sick. Who knows how these things work?

Anyway, on top of the usual torments of adolescence—the raging hormones, the problems with authority—I had the extra burdens of suddenly being "the man of the house." In some ways, frankly, I was exemplary in the role. A model son. A combination fix-it man and dorm monitor.

In other ways I really screwed it up.

I guess I *had* to screw it up, to give myself more slack than the system thought acceptable. If I didn't, my head would have exploded from the pressure. Or—just as bad—I would have ended up bitter and resentful in my later life.

Typically, the place I messed up was in school. When my father died, we moved from Greenwich to Bethesda, Maryland. I went through the small death of leaving my friends, my junior high rock band. I entered my new school with no pals and a lousy attitude.

I'd been placed in accelerated classes, but since I did no homework, I got kicked out of them. Regular classes bored me to rage, so I started playing hooky. Your basic downward spiral.

I fell in with the wrong crowd. I started doing some knucklehead things, like petty shoplifting. Even now this embarrasses me, but hey, this isn't a résumé, this is life.

Life is complicated, and rich, and anyone who claims he never did anything bad is either a liar or a total nerd. Even St. Augustine stole pears as a young man. It's how he discovered the anguish of a guilty conscience and came to understand the supreme value of a clear one.

Besides, one of the peaceful things about being near the end of life is that I don't have to flinch from mistakes I've made along the way. Truthfully, my mistakes don't seem to have mattered very much. They were dumb, not evil, and dumb is part of every life.

Looking back, I realize that at fourteen, fifteen, I was in a total fog. The stupor that descended on me the night my father died had never really lifted. I told myself I was in charge of my fate, *deciding* things, but much of the time I didn't know what I was doing, or why. And, of course, like every befuddled adolescent, I imagined that no one but me had ever undergone such frustration and confusion.

But here's the part that may seem surprising: Even at the nadir of my helplessness and floundering, I always sort of knew that things would turn out fine. Beyond my short-term misery lay a long-term optimism that never really flagged.

Two things, I think, explain this paradox. One is the nature of the times I lived in. The other is the amazing character of my mother.

In the middle 1960s, the old rules were just beginning to be stretched. In retrospect, there's something meek and even quaint about the things that seemed radical then. The Beatles' hair covered their ears. They wore sports jackets without lapels. These things passed for scandalous subversions.

Still, the times were loosening up. Like most fifties kids, I'd been raised in fear of the dreaded "black mark"—the single mistake that would be indelibly written into my "permanent record" and that would utterly ruin my chances of success in later life. By the middle sixties that "permanent record" nonsense was beginning to be seen as the manipulative joke that it was.

Of course kids made mistakes. Of course they experimented—with smoking, with sex, with drugs, with whatever form of rebellion was in vogue at the time; how else did we learn? Who of our generation except for some fibbing politicians and a handful of goody-goody misfits would brag that he never inhaled?

And of course most of us would survive our errors and outgrow our experiments and end up as responsible adults— eventually. In the meantime, people of our generation seemed to agree that it was more important to live fully than to live in a straight line. I never doubted that even in a short life there would be time to get back on track, to regain momentum, to make amends. Having this faith—*living by* this faith—was one of the ways in which my generation has been so fortunate.

But social changes alone wouldn't have saved this floundering kid if not for my mother's being rock-solid on the home front.

I realize that so far I've hardly talked about my mother. That's because her effect on me has been so thorough and so subtle that I hardly know what to say about it. If my father, in many ways, shaped my life, my mother has been the one who saved my life. My father had a dramatic impact by dying; my mother has had a gentler impact by enduring. (She endures still, God bless her, at the age of seventy-eight.)

I'm incredibly proud of my mother. I think of her as a truly evolved woman. Which is my shorthand way of saying strong, adaptable, always finding something good in what was difficult, always looking forward.

At the time of my father's death, my mother was a typical housewife. She shopped for groceries, cooked meals, smoothed down her sons' cowlicks. In practical matters she seemed to be a total airhead. Knew nothing about money. Couldn't balance a checkbook.

Until she had to. Then my mother revealed that, all along, she'd had impressive resources and versatility. She was so smart, in fact, that it cost her nothing, during my father's lifetime, to hang back and let him be the smart one.

Now she went back to college, finished an interrupted education, and earned her teaching credentials. Somehow she provided for three boys on a grade-school teacher's salary. Our homes were modest but she always managed to settle us in nice neighborhoods. If there were financial strains, she grew ever more skillful at keeping them hidden. I swear I don't know how she did all that.

It taught me something about men and women, though. Men tend to be the ones who yammer on about making big changes in their lives. But women deal much better with the changes when they happen. Men bellow; women adapt.

Anyway, of all the things my mother did for me, one of the most impressive was that, even in our straitened circumstances, she managed to rescue me from truancy and self-defeat, by sending me to a wonderful prep school called Loomis.

Again, I don't know how she managed it financially. But I think that, in her wisdom, my mother figured out something that I wouldn't grasp for many years: By goofing off in adolescence, I was in some way paying myself back for the part of childhood I'd been gypped out of. I acted feisty and independent, but largely I was frightened and confused; what I really craved was structure and safety.

Loomis provided that. You've heard of the three-strikes rule? Loomis had a one-strike rule. One major screw-up and you're history. I loved the clarity of it.

So I didn't screw up at Loomis because I couldn't screw up. I may have been a bit of a mess but I wasn't downright stupid. Even then I knew the difference between a mistake and a disaster.

◆◆◆

IN THINKING about the deep discomfort of adolescence, it occurs to me that the pain comes from this:

You find yourself on the cusp of something new and unknown—adulthood—and deep down inside you fear you aren't ready for it. You don't know the game. You don't like the rules. You're afraid of being overwhelmed, humiliated. The greater your fear, the greater your resentment at being put in that circumstance.

It dawns on me now that a terminal illness also goes through a kind of adolescence, and for a very similar reason.

Again you're on the brink of a new phase. Again there's the confusion and fear and anger that go with doubts about your readiness. Only now the next phase is death.

For me, the "adolescence" of my illness came in the spring of 2000.

As I've said, I was first diagnosed near the end of 1998. My first surgery was deemed a great success. I was told that if I made it past the one-year mark with no return of cancer I was almost certainly home free. I believed in that prognosis. Why wouldn't I?

At the beginning I had monthly checkups. On the way to those appointments, I knocked on a lot of wood. I was nervous, and I had no problem yielding to my superstitions. You could also say that I was beginning to remember how to pray.

I was doing well. My checkups became quarterly. I cruised past six months, nine months. I had a clean one-year exam.

After it, I took my wife in my arms and cried for joy. I don't think I'd realized quite how frightened I'd been all year. Now it all poured out of me.

I felt reborn. I don't mean spiritually here. I mean literally, physically. My body was mine again. My skin felt new. I looked in the mirror and saw a still-young, undaunted face. I'd dodged the bullet. I'd beaten cancer.

Except I hadn't.

At the eighteen-month exam, the malignancy reappeared. This was shocking, inexplicable, unfair. I'd endured my year in purgatory, obeyed the terms of my probation. They'd *told* me I would be okay. Why was the game suddenly changed again?

I was furious—as baffled and angry as any adolescent knocking his head against a hostile and stubborn reality. In my private thoughts, I started looking for someone to blame.

My big-shot surgeon had messed up, let a speck of something deadly fall off the scalpel. The oncologists had lied about my chances. The lab technicians blew it when checking for clean margins. I was mad at everyone. My anger may have been childish; it may also have been necessary. Either way, it didn't change a thing.

I had cancer again. And here's a sorry bit of math: Having cancer twice is way more than twice as bad as having cancer once. Recurrence is the disease's war cry, the sure signal that the stakes have been raised to nothing less than life or death.

Now I needed radiation, chemo. The treatments would make me far sicker than the disease had managed to so far.

Faced with the debilitating therapies, I could no longer hide behind my phony ulcer story. I would finally be outed as a cancer patient. My kids would know how sick I was.

Friends would feel sorry for me. I can hardly express how much I hated that part. But it led me to reexamine the depth of some of my "friendships." How can I put this? I've been incredibly fortunate to have had a few close buddies, guys I love and who love me back, people I can confide in. People from whom I would hide nothing—not even cancer.

Then there's a larger group that I've hung around with because of shared work and comparable economic standing. I genuinely like and admire most of these people. But are we *friends*, or did we just hang around to feel like winners, alpha guys together? If the friendships were more substantial than that, why did I want to hide from these guys now that I was weakened, diminished? Why was I so embarrassed?

These feelings were excruciating. Just like the social uncertainties of adolescence.

So off I went into this next phase of my illness. Outwardly, I think I behaved well enough. "Appropriately," whatever that means exactly in a situation like this. I was a grown-up, after all. But my spirit kicked and screamed like that of a cornered teenager.

For much of my life I'd had a favorite motto, a personal mantra derived from skiing, but with application off the slopes as well: *No one gets hurt in the air*. As long as I was soaring, my twists and turns and even my contortions couldn't really harm me. But now I was faced with something that clearly threatened to bring me down to earth, and I was painfully aware that I was largely powerless to avoid the crash.

6

SOMEHOW OR OTHER, Loomis made a decent student out of me.

Two things contributed to this. They may sound contradictory, but they aren't. First, I discovered that I actually enjoyed learning; loved it, in fact. Second, I came to the very useful realization that school is basically a game, and, as with any game, it's more fun if you win.

The thorny attitude of my earlier adolescence didn't go away, but I found ways to make it work for me rather than against me. And that might be as close as I can get to defining the process of becoming a successful adult.

This is something I've noticed again and again in life: There's a fine line between adolescent anger and frustration and the kind of drive and determination that make for success in later life, especially in business. What had been mere combativeness can ripen into what I think of as creative irreverence. It's really just a matter of managing the energy—and, frankly, the insecurity—and funneling it in productive ways.

Anyway, I did well enough at Loomis that I was accepted for college at Columbia. Now, Columbia is a fine school, but if I thought I was in for a top-notch, Ivy League education, I was wrong. Fact is, there was not a great deal of classroom learning going on there in those years. The Vietnam protests were at their height. Buildings were occupied. Classes were canceled.

It was uncool to admit this, but I was deeply disappointed about all that. I wanted the education I'd signed on for. My family had scrimped to send me to a first-tier school and I didn't take their sacrifices lightly. I had a partial scholarship on which the clock was ticking, whether classes were held or not. Moreover, as part of my hurry-up philosophy, I wanted to graduate in three years.

So I was in a bit of a bind. As a card-carrying hippie I was sympathetic to demonstrators of every stripe, but as an ambitious young man with his own agenda I resented that they were protesting on my precious time.

I was against the war, of course. It was a cynical, dishonest escapade and it never should have happened. But let me make a confession, which I believe also applies to a large proportion of my contemporaries. My political convictions were not especially profound, and in fact were pretty thin. First and foremost, I was against the war because I was intent on preserving my own young butt.

That may not sound very noble, but far from being ashamed of it, I'm proud of its reasonableness. What is saner than not wanting to die at nineteen years of age? What is more rational than declining to be a sacrificial lamb? If everyone felt that way, the world would be a far less violent place.

I went to my fair share of antiwar demonstrations. But again, let me be candid about my less-than-lofty motives. I believed in the cause, sure. But it's also true that demonstrations were a great place to meet girls. Everybody knew that. Demonstrations were gigantic parties. They often featured live music, generally marijuana was passed around, and everyone was friends, just by the fact of showing up.

Thank God my generation had those rituals, those almost primitive experiences of bonding with a huge, like-minded group. The occasion for these enormous get-togethers was secondary. The main thing was just that they happened. They gave us a sense of ourselves as a force in the world. And each of us, individually, could carry away some morsel of that power.

It's funny, in a way, because I think of myself as a very active individual; I'm proud of what I've *done*. But when I think back on those massive hippie gatherings, I realize it doesn't matter what I did, but only that I was *there*, part of a great huddle of humanity. As individuals, who knows how much we really had in common, or even if we would have liked one another for very long. But that's not the point. The point is that we were truly joined in those moments, linked to something bigger than our own precious egos. At the end of my life, as I try to sum up what was valuable and what was busywork, I still cherish that vanished sense of community, of connection. My life would have been poorer without it.

Music was a big part of the community, of course. When I think about the high points of my college years, music is what I think of first.

Since classes were so often canceled, and since I needed extra money, I started looking for work as a studio musician or a fill-in guy for groups that needed a keyboard player. That's how I ended up as the only white guy in a twenty-six-piece Motown group. For someone who admired black music as much as I did, this was an experience almost beyond the reach of fantasy. We played at a lot of outdoor concerts and rallies. We also had some gigs at the legendary Apollo Theater, up in Harlem. Once we opened for James Brown, the Godfather of Soul himself. I played an organ called the Hammond B-3—a wailing, screaming percussive instrument designed for shaking walls. And the walls *did* shake at the Apollo. The energy was astounding.

Hanging around the Columbia dorms, I also jammed occasionally with some fellows whose approach to the music fascinated me. Ahead of their time, they were already, in 1968 or so, taking a retro, campy approach to rock. They sang doo-wop. They did lampoons of sappy teenage-death songs.

Just my luck, after I stopped sitting in with them they solidified the group, turned pro, appeared at Woodstock, and got fairly famous. The group's name was Sha-Na-Na.

I don't consider myself a nostalgic person. In fact I've always had a certain horror of nostalgia. I've always looked ahead, not back. I've always felt that there are few sadder things in life than peaking too soon, then wasting decades in reliving the supposed glory years of youth.

Even now, as my body is failing and I'm dying, I continue to believe there will be moments—alone with my thoughts, or talking with a friend, or in the company of my wife and kids— that will be richer and more meaningful than anything that has gone before. I really believe that.

At the same time, I can now look back at my youth with a kind of detached affection—as if it were not my own life I was recalling, but that of an old buddy with whom I'd drifted out of touch. And I can acknowledge, with serenity, that there were episodes of vigor and joy and off-the-charts excitement that will never come again.

One of those episodes was an outdoor concert that Sha-Na-Na played in the Columbia quad.

It was a time of great tension on campus and in the racially troubled surrounding neighborhood. The school administration—who didn't really get it, obviously—thought that a super-loud rock concert might be a way to calm things down. So they had a stage built in front of Butler Library, and they opened the quad to fifty thousand people.

It was a hot night. The band played for hours and hours. The sound couldn't escape—it just bounced off the buildings and fed on itself. Having some familiarity with the group, I could tell what they'd rehearsed and when they were just winging it. It didn't matter. It was all great. People sang along till they were hoarse. They swayed together and pressed against the stage. Strangers were suddenly friends. People met each other's eyes and were suddenly in love.

Thinking back to that concert, I understand why young people believe that they will live forever.

Here's an eighteen-, nineteen-year-old kid. He's full to bursting with music and libido. He's surrounded by dancing and noise. He barely knows what it is to be tired. How can that pumped-up kid imagine an end of youth and strength, how could he envision ever feeling any way but good?

How could such vitality exhaust itself in the eye-blink of a few short decades?

◆ ◆ ◆

FOR SOMEONE accustomed to feeling good, to taking vitality for granted, the ravages of current cancer therapies come as a horrible affront.

Chemo is poison. Radiation is like some science-fiction death ray. These are violent and frankly desperate ways of treating a disease.

I don't claim to be an expert or a scientist, but having been around the whole wide world of cancer treatments, there's one extremely confident prediction I will make: Before too much longer, our current modes of treating the disease will come to seem as barbaric and primitive as bloodletting. (Remember, bloodletting "cured" some people too.) The future lies in more targeted therapies that won't decimate the entire body in the name of attacking a few offensive cells.

Anyway, I see no point in detailing the physical trials and humiliations that are part of cancer treatment; there's nothing redemptive or even interesting about nausea and profound exhaustion. But I do think there might be value in regarding the role that treatment played in my evolving state of mind—in the complicated dance that my disease and I were doing.

I said a while back that the recurrence of my cancer corresponded to the adolescence of the illness. Well, adolescence is when a person feels most totally defined by his body. There are so many new pleasures to discover: the pleasure of sex, the pleasure of sports, the sheer animal joy of feeling strong and of growing stronger. Sure, there's awkwardness and anxiety as well; but basically, when you're a vigorous and healthy adolescent, you find it's pretty great to have a body.

In the "adolescence" of my sickness, I didn't yet think very much about what cancer—and, more specifically, its treatment—

was doing to (and for) my psyche and my soul; I fixed on what it was doing to my physical self. And since it was doing nothing but bad things, I felt frustrated and wretched.

I started casting about for ways to feel less bad. I read a fair amount of philosophy. And I noticed something that intrigued me, because it cut across so many different lines of thought.

Whether you read the ancient Greeks, or the Zen masters, or the New Testament, everybody seems to agree that the soul is *imprisoned* by the body, and that only death can set it free. The body, at best, is an encumbrance and a nuisance; at worst, it's a sink of depravity and a beastly obstacle to salvation.

As a young and healthy man—in the midst of the sexual revolution, no less—I wouldn't have bought that at all.

It would have struck me as prudish, bloodless, half dead already. Thank you very much, but I didn't *want* a soul without a body. I was a sensualist, and proud of it.

I felt then, and still believe, that neglecting the physical side of life is as much of a sin as neglecting the spiritual. Either way, you're wasting part of what it is to be a human being.

Here's the rub: It's the physical side that fades, that becomes increasingly problematical and is vulnerable to decay. In the face of illness and debility, there *does* come a point when the body is the enemy, and being free of it seems like nothing but a blessed release.

I accept that now. I didn't accept it then, during the adolescent phase of my cancer. And because I didn't accept it, I suffered.

Like everybody else, I suppose, I've known a fair range of bad feelings in my life. I've known worry, anger, loss. But during my early regimens of cancer treatment, when my bodily vigor was being sapped and my sense of strength was being mocked, I had glimpses of something I'd never confronted before, something I'd thought was utterly foreign to my temperament: depression.

Maybe the feeling was a purely chemical reaction to the treatments. Maybe it was an emotional response to my loss of control. Maybe it was the shadow cast by fear. Whatever it was, it was grim. I felt hope ebbing away. It wasn't just that I was losing the battle, but that I was having ever greater difficulty finding the heart to fight at all.

One day, when my body was wracked and my head ached and my spirits were at their lowest, I said to my wife: "I just don't see the point."

Now, my wife Laura is as supportive and kind as a person could possibly be. I'm in awe of her gentleness. But in that moment she was something other than tender; she was absolutely fierce.

Fierce on my behalf—and, I think, on her own. She still had the determination that I was having such a hard time mustering. She still saw value in the struggle. She wasn't about to let me wallow. She already had enough burdens; she didn't want to cater to someone who had given up.

"So *find* one!" she declared.

I was so surprised by her vehemence that I lost my train of thought. I said, "Huh?"

"You don't see the point?" she said. "Find a point!"

Looking back, I realize just how important that brief but intense conversation was.

It turned me around. This was not instantaneous. There was no lightning bolt. But Laura's fire somehow entered into me. I became more able to accept the obvious fact that my life had changed and would continue to change.

Not that I took it lying down. Life was taking back many of the pleasures it had given me, and I missed them. The miraculous loans of strength and physical ease were coming due, and the payback cost me dearly. I knew only too well what I was losing to my illness; the great challenge now lay in discovering what I was being given in return.

Finding the point *became* the point. That was the realm in which I still had everything to gain.

7

I DON'T KNOW who said this first, but there's a lot of wisdom in it: *A problem that can be fixed by money . . . is not a problem.*

It's an inconvenience, maybe. A discomfort. A glitch. And money is great for smoothing over those sorts of unpleasantness.

But when it comes to a real problem, like cancer, money turns out to be surprisingly useless. With money, the doctors might fuss over you a little more, you can die in a nicer room, but if you're terminal, you're terminal. I don't mean to sound flip or overly harsh, that's just how it is.

To put it another way, if you've got your health, you can always make some money. But all the dough in the world can't buy back your health.

Everybody knows that, right? But here's an odd thing I've noticed about people: If you put aside what they *say* and look at how people actually *live*, you'd have to conclude that they believe the opposite. People exhaust themselves to advance at their jobs. Business travelers eat appallingly unhealthy food at airports, then drink too much to wind down from the day. They go without exercise; they go without sleep.

Now, I'm either the best or the worst person to pass along this lesson, because I was guilty of violating it myself. But isn't it clear that the person who compromises his health in the name of making money is cutting himself a really lousy deal?

This is not a knock against money. I'm not, at this late stage, denying that I'm an avid capitalist, or that I'm proud of my material success. I'm just trying to achieve some perspective. In the scale of good things, money comes way after health, and after family, and after friends. Of course, it's easier to say all that once one *has* some money. In fact, maybe the single best thing about having money is that it makes money seem a great deal less important.

Which reminds me of a sixties myth I'd like to dispel.

When people wax nostalgic about how great the sixties were, one of the claims they make is that back then no one cared about money. Well, I don't think that's exactly accurate. Fewer people *worried* about money, because we all had the unspoken confidence that money would come. How can I put it? It was as if history itself had given my whole generation a gigantic trust fund. We didn't deserve this; we didn't *not* deserve it either; it just fell our way, an inheritance from the amazing post–World War II economic boom and the unprecedented prosperity of the American Century.

Let me tell a story about my first inkling that I had a knack for making dough, that money would come when needed. It was the fall of 1971. I was still at Columbia, and it had become clear to me that my partial scholarship, and the help my mother could provide, and the little bit of money I made from music and from summer jobs, were not going to be enough to get me through the rest of college. I was seriously afraid that I would have to quit.

So I formed a plan. I'd apply for one of those low-cost student loans, take the money, and invest it. Understand, I knew almost nothing about investing. But someone had told me that orange juice futures offered a great opportunity. This wasn't rocket science. If bad weather in California or Florida or Mexico or Brazil cut into the size of the orange crop, the futures jumped in value. So I plunked down $1,870—a lot of borrowed money!—on orange juice futures.

Almost immediately, the value of my contracts started going down. And kept going down. And I thought about something I'd conveniently overlooked before: What if there was great weather all over the citrus belt? What if 1971 was a banner year for OJ? Good news for Tropicana. Bad news for me. I'd lose my shirt.

I worried. I fretted. I was literally sick over it. I quickly came to understand that I took no pleasure from the suspense of gambling. I neglected my schoolwork and started hanging around the broker's office, wondering when to cut my losses.

Then, during the week before my contracts were to expire, there was a freak freeze in Florida. The OJ market panicked and spiked. I sold my futures and pocketed a profit of $7,490.

Was I smart? No. Was I lucky? Absolutely. Dumb lucky.

The point is that the money was there to be made. It was just a matter of getting into the game. Even a know-nothing hippie like me could do it.

There's a coda to this story that I want to tell, in part because it shows how wildly naïve I was, but also because it demonstrates the essential benevolence of the times I lived in.

With the money I made in OJ, I repaid my loan and took care of my tuition. Amazingly, I had enough cash left over to buy a somewhat beat-up secondhand Porsche. The day I bought it I drove it all over Manhattan. Up the FDR Drive, down the West Side Highway. I was in heaven. That night I parked it on the street in front of my dorm, in Morningside Heights.

This was truly dumb. I awoke to find my Porsche sitting on its belly on the asphalt. The wheels had been stolen. I'd had the car one day and it was trashed.

New wheels and assorted repairs used up the last of my windfall profits. But at least I'd learned where not to park. I needed a safe space. However, I was broke again—back to my usual mode. A Manhattan garage was out of the question.

I got out a New York City transit map. What I was looking for was a subway line, convenient to Columbia, that ended in a wealthy neighborhood. That's how I discovered Riverdale, a beautiful area way up in the Bronx, perched on bluffs above the Hudson. Riverdale was like a piece of Dutchess County within the city limits.

I drove up there, parked the car on a tree-lined street of gracious homes, and started knocking on the doors of complete strangers, asking them if they had extra room in their driveway or garage. Not surprisingly, people looked at me like I was crazy—a student-hippie-bum trying to stash a fancy car. A couple of people slammed their doors in my face. One lady threatened to call the cops.

The only surprising part is that one woman didn't slam the door.

She was the classiest lady I'd ever seen—perfect gray hair, informal but elegant clothes. She reminded me of Katharine Hepburn. When she heard I was a student at Columbia, she invited me in for tea; she was genuinely curious about the unrest there, about what young people were thinking. And so we got to talking. Her name was Mrs. Simon. As in Simon and Schuster. She told me I just had to meet her two daughters, Lucy and Carly. After a while, they came in. I was instantly smitten with Carly, who was not only gorgeous but had, even then, an indefinable specialness about her. Star-quality, I guess.

Carly had less than zero interest in me. She saw me, I suppose, as exactly what I was: a green kid who'd shown up at her house to beg a favor, a nobody with chutzpah.

Which is fine. I *was* a nobody. But at least I was a nobody who believed that wonderful things could happen, that the world

I lived in was benign and would give me at least some of what I hoped for.

During the rest of my tenure at Columbia, my old Porsche stayed in the Simons' garage. For fifteen cents I could ride the Number 1 train up to visit it. If I was lucky, I might catch a glimpse of Carly. Then I'd drive around Riverdale awhile, pretending I belonged there.

◆ ◆ ◆

"*FIND A POINT!*" my wife had insisted, when I was in the depths of my funk, when chemo was sapping my strength, when I was knocking my head against the hard truth that my world was beginning to contract, my options starting to diminish.

It was a tall order. I'd never been a very introspective person. My energies had generally been directed outward, toward adventures in the wider world. I wasn't someone who sat in his room, thinking deep thoughts. I was the guy in the dinged-up Porsche, revving high, jumping lanes, out there trying to *accomplish* something. And accomplishment, for me, had always meant a victory that could be measured against some outside standard—a grade in school, a score in a lacrosse game, a deal in business—something that could be recorded on a report card or a balance sheet.

I was accustomed to being in control—not just of my own destiny, but of complicated enterprises. Now I wasn't even in control of my digestion. My schedule was built around medical appointments, my vigor rose and fell as a function of foreign chemicals pumped into my body.

So where was I supposed to find something to feel good about, some realm where I could still feel strong and hopeful? The answer now seems obvious, but for me it was the hardest place to accept: that realm was my mind.

My frame of mind was something I could still control. Doing so would be a sort of victory I was not accustomed to valuing—a totally inward, private victory—but a legitimate accomplishment nevertheless. I resolved to control my own discomforts, to rise above them if I possibly could. In so doing, I came to understand the deep truth that, while pain may be unavoidable, suffering is largely optional.

Maybe a Zen master can actually conquer pain. Unfortunately, that's way beyond me. When I hurt, I hurt. But it's the *attitude* toward the pain that makes all the difference. Pain can make you thoroughly miserable, or pain can just be pain. The trick, I've realized, is to confine it to the body and not let it infect the mind.

Or, if you prefer, the soul.

This is another of the words that was not even in my vocabulary till recently; and to be honest, I'm not even sure exactly what I mean by it. But that's okay—I'm no theologian. Besides, I mistrust rigid definitions. They're the beginning of dogma, and dogma is the start of narrow-mindedness.

I have a *feeling* about what soul is, if not the words to pin it down precisely. I think of soul as something that includes the mind but goes beyond the mind; something that sums up what a person has tried to be in life but that also goes beyond the individual. And soul, I believe, endures after death. Can I rationally justify that belief? No. Does it bother me that I can't? Not anymore.

In any case, the soul is something that should be outside the reach of physical pain. Pain, I realize now, is one of the things that urges us to separate the soul from the body. I'm not being flippant if I put it in business terms; those terms just make a lot of sense to me. The soul and the body are like long-term business partners. For some decades they make a brilliant team. They each bring something essential to the party of life; they really complement each other. But when things head south for the body, the soul must either be dragged down or take steps to dissolve the partnership.

There's a next level where the soul can go, and the body can't. Not that dissolving a partnership is ever easy. But the alternative is even worse. Let the soul be sullied by the complaints of the body, and you've lost not only in one of life's arenas, but two.

I promised myself, and promised Laura, that I would try my absolute hardest not to let that happen. Bodily pain would be the body's problem. I'd concentrate on learning how to keep my mind unclouded, my soul free to soar.

8

I<small>F</small> I <small>HAVE ANYTHING AT ALL</small> to teach about life, it probably comes down to these two simple but far-reaching notions:

Recognizing the difference between a dumb risk and a smart one, and

Understanding when you need to change direction, and having the guts to do it.

So many of the big decisions that define a life—whether in business, or in starting a family, or even in facing a terminal disease—come down to managing these two ideas.

I can clearly remember the first time my own life made a high-stakes U-turn. I remember the fear and self-doubt that preceded the big move. Was I being a jerk? Was I ruining my life?

Even more vividly, I remember the invigoration that came after.

What happened was this. True to my hurry-up philosophy, I'd graduated Columbia in three years and enrolled directly in a master's program there. My field was international relations—which, in my naïveté, I imagined had to do with things like promoting world peace and encouraging the progress of the poorer nations. As I moved through the program, however, it became clear that my youthful ideals were woefully out of step with how the world actually worked. Several credits shy of a master's, I could no longer dodge the deflating conclusion that my degree would qualify me for nothing but a job with the World Bank or the IMF.

It so happened that I detest those organizations. Beyond their high-flown rhetoric, their real mandate is to foster a climate in which the biggest companies and banks from the richest nations can continue to make money, generally at the expense of the poorer countries. I wasn't about to dedicate my life to *that*.

So I packed up and left.

My professors were mystified. My mother was deeply disappointed. And I don't blame her. If my own kids pulled a stunt like that, I'd certainly try to talk them out of it. The voice of parental reason would say: Finish the degree, get the credential, *then* decide if it's really what you want.

Sound advice. Guidance-counselor wisdom. But it looks very different when it's your own life.

I was going purely on instinct. I ran a gut-check, and followed its dictates. Looking back, I think I must have had some rudimentary understanding of how people get trapped in life, how staying on a track can kill, one easy day at a time.

It would have been easy to finish that degree—easier than bolting. With the degree in hand, it would have been easier for me to land a job with one of the status quo watchdogs than with anybody else. Once I had the job, it would have been easier to amend my own beliefs than to change the organization.

Thus, by increments so exquisitely gradual that they might have passed unnoticed, I could have ended up being totally untrue to myself and living a life I hated. Twenty years later, I might have had a closet full of suits, a passport full of visas, and an irreparable feeling that I'd really blown it.

No thanks. Call me irresponsible, but I think it's better to zig and zag before the first foot is in the trap.

So I hit the road, literally. I bought an ancient, UPS-style, Step-Van truck, and, mostly with lumber pilfered from various construction sites, fitted it out as a mobile home worthy of Ken Kesey's Magic Bus. I took a girlfriend and a buddy, and we left the East Coast and headed for the Rocky Mountains. Mission: Ski as much as possible on practically no money.

At the time, we congratulated ourselves on being highly original; in retrospect, though, so much of what happened was absolutely typical of the period. We thought we were exercising absolute freedom; but freedom, I've learned, is never absolute. There's always a context. Our options were defined and our choices steered by a sort of generational zeitgeist.

Far from feeling deflated about this, I get a kick out of it. It pleases me to know that I have sung along with my times, that I've vibrated with the frequencies that were thrumming through the air. As I've said, I make no claim of being special. But I jumped with both feet into what was going on.

Living in what was called, simply, the Green Truck, we drove when we wanted to drive, and stopped when we wanted to stop. Most nights we spent at closed gas stations. We'd pull up near the Coke machine, unplug it, and stick in our own two-hundred-foot extension cord. We had light, heat, and music, on someone else's electric bill.

This was theft, but forgive me for feeling no remorse whatsoever. It didn't feel like stealing; it felt like cozying up to the breast of a kind and generous world. We were learning the hugely valuable lesson that fun and money are two different things. And, as I would come to understand later, wealth is a great deal more enjoyable if you've already taught yourself that you can have a good time without it.

Not that life in the Green Truck was without its difficulties and minor heartbreaks that seemed major at the time. There were moods. There was road weariness. Inevitably, my girlfriend segued into a liaison with my buddy. I certainly had my share of youthful jealousy and pining. But that's okay. We were kids and it was the early seventies. There were other girlfriends, and other buddies—an ever-changing cast of brief but sincere and rollicking friendships.

It was so easy to make friends then. People met on the road, smoked a joint or had a couple beers, and were soon discussing the meaning of life. Or climbing mountains together. Or telling each other their dreams. Or laughing hysterically, tears streaming, at things that maybe weren't even all that funny.

If I had the time, I could tell a hundred stories about the Green Truck phase. I could rhapsodize about the first astonishing view of the mountains rising from the plains, or about the blue smell of fresh snow at eleven thousand feet. But if I had to take that whole bundle of experience and distill it down to one key point, what I'd say is this: The time spent in the Green Truck was the closest I'd come to living entirely in the present. I didn't plan. I didn't worry. I had no particular destination beyond the place I'd park that night. I was aimless, and proud of it. I lived with the intensity of *here*. I enjoyed the excitement and serenity of *now*. This was a privilege whose full value I'm not sure I recognized at the time.

I did recognize it, though, when, after several bustling and achieving decades—decades dedicated to the building of a future—I finally felt the freedom once again of being entirely rooted in the here and now.

That happened when I accepted the fact that I was dying.

♦ ♦ ♦

HERE'S A PARADOX. I'll tell you up front that I can't resolve it, but neither, to the best of my knowledge, can anybody else.

Commentators on human happiness, from the Buddha to the latest psychobabbling guru, are always harping on the importance of living in the present moment. But, unless you're content to spend your life sitting under a tree and begging alms, that simply isn't possible. To be a functioning human being you've got to be concerned about the future.

Kids learn in grade school that present actions have future consequences. Cause and effect. If A, then B. The "smart" kids are the ones who grasp that right away. The ones who dawdle in the present are thought of as dummies or hopeless daydreamers.

In business, the whole idea is to figure out what *will* happen, and to prepare for it before anybody else does. The present hardly exists, except as a launchpad for the future. You've got to plan. Which is another way of saying *you've got to worry*.

Worrying, then, becomes practically the defining trait of the responsible adult. Maturity becomes the willingness to sacrifice the *now* on the altar of the *later*.

Maybe this is necessary in order to "succeed" in life. But I can hardly imagine how to assess the cost of it—in enjoyment, in peace of mind, maybe even in bodily health. For decades, as a responsible grown-up and ambitious businessman, I lived largely in the future. Everything was a strategy, a plan, a scheme. The present went by in a blur as I raced toward someplace else.

Not that I wasn't enjoying myself. I was having a blast. Business was exciting and fulfilling. With that satisfaction as a background, I totally cherished the time when I wasn't working. There were wonderful family vacations, fabulous weekends with friends, moments of great joy with my wife.

But—how can I put it?—I often felt like I was merely visiting the present, dropping in for precious interludes. The norm was to be chasing things that were always up ahead. I was so immersed in the future that I barely noticed I was short-selling the current hours as they passed. And I might never have thought about it if I hadn't gotten sick.

Once my unproductive anger about this lousy break started to subside, I began thinking less about what cancer was doing to me and more about what it was doing *for* me. And I realized something sort of wonderful. Cancer was giving me the opportunity to live more attentively, more wholly in the moment. It was letting me be as free and as focused on the present as I'd been in the heyday of the Green Truck.

Once I understood that the disease was killing me, I realized that, for most practical purposes, I no longer had a future. I had some indefinite amount of time ahead of me—but that's not exactly the same thing. Future implies progress, choices, uncertainty. For better or worse, what lay ahead for me was no longer uncertain.

No future. If that notion is surreal and terrifying, it is also vastly liberating. I'd be leaving soon; things that happened no longer mattered very much to me. Consequences? Don't expect a dying person to worry too damn much about consequences. Parking tickets? Throw 'em away! Today's business headlines? Who cares?

My family, of course, had a future, and making provision for them was a sacred and joyful obligation. Beyond that, I was home free. I had nothing but the present, and I resolved to make the most of it.

I promised myself that I wouldn't have a bad day for the rest of my life. If someone was wasting my time, I'd excuse myself and walk away. If a situation bothered me or refused to get resolved, I'd shrug and move on. I'd squander no energy on petty annoyances, poison no minutes with useless regret. I'd play music at any hour of the day or night. I'd make a point of noticing the smell of the air, the shifting light on the mountains.

In recent months, on more than one occasion, one of my kids has walked into my study, and said, "Hi, Dad. What're you smiling about?" The funny part is that I haven't been able to tell them. I couldn't remember what I'd been thinking, or even if I'd been thinking anything at all. Had I been reminiscing? Fantasizing? Watching a hawk land in a tree above the pond? Or just sitting there, inhabiting a moment, basking in the pleasure of the present? All I can say for sure is that I was oddly, simply happy.

THE READINESS IS ALL.

—Shakespeare, *Hamlet*

♦ ♦ ♦

PETER IS DETERMINED to live until he dies.

This expression—to live until one's death—is of course an old one, a cliché that's stuck around because it points to a fundamental truth. But I'd never thought below the surface of the words until observing Peter—seeing the stubborn and exalted contrast between his physical failing and the richness of his days.

Peter's body is dying by increments. As with the most sadistic kinds of torture, the hallmark of his disease is its relentless gradualness.

Tumors slowly and inexorably grow. Blockages develop; stressed systems struggle to function. Peter's store of resilience is inevitably paid out, like a losing gambler's stack of chips. His pain increases; the periods without pain become ever more fleeting oases. The body slowly fades.

But Peter's spirit will have none of that.

He refuses to accept the waning of intensity and joy. He insists that his wonderful moments shall continue. If the cost of those moments is exhaustion, he's more than willing to exhaust himself. There's a kind of ecstasy in flinging himself against the wall of physical limits, waging war against the ultimate fatigue. He will, as they say, live until he dies.

Here is what the Barton family did on Easter morning of 2002:

At around five A.M., Laura woke the kids. Peter was already in the kitchen, throwing together a breakfast that he himself couldn't eat. By five-thirty, breath steaming in the darkness, the family had piled into a car and was heading west, toward the foothills of the Rockies.

The air got ever brisker as they broke free of the city and began to climb the mountains. A late moon made crisp silhouettes of spruce trees and ponderosa pines; stars still burned above the snowcaps of the Front Range. The hum of their tires was the only sound along the empty roads.

Just as the seam of the horizon was beginning to show in the east, they stopped at a small clearing where a huge hot-air balloon was being inflated. Its brightly colored panels seemed to drink in the pale light; it was as if the light itself would give the craft its buoyancy.

The Bartons climbed into the gondola, Peter lugging his ever-present IV backpack. The pilot fired up the hot-air jets. The lines were released and the balloon lifted off. It coasted above the treetops, over plummeting canyons and vast swaths of untouched snow. Between hissing bursts of bright-blue flame, an ancient silence reigned. Peter put his arms around his family as they floated to the top of the world.

Finally they rose above the level of the highest peaks. To the west and north and south, the Rockies arched and writhed in their epic corrugations; to the east, the Great Plains stretched away forever. And then the sun came up.

Peter told me later: "The snow turned pink. The granite was an amazing yellow-gray. The Plains, in a heartbeat, went from black to this honey-like gold. The mountains looked brand-new, like they'd sprung up overnight . . .

"That was my sunrise service. There in the mountains, my spiritual home. Flying with my family, looking out on a million miles of just-created world."

I looked closely at Peter as he told me this. His features were serene; his eyes were wide with wonder. And I thought: Is this the same man who, just a few short months ago, would bristle at a mention of the spiritual—who would grow impatient and embarrassed at any suggestion that he was a reflective person?

Clearly, Peter was going through a remarkable evolution, a journey that was accelerated and intensified by the daily experience of being ill. As life grew more difficult and more painful, death seemed ever more a mercy and a consummation. It was ever more important to Peter to prepare himself for the inevitable crossing-over, to die with dignity and grace.

But that was no small task. It took enormous concentration, and a letting go of lifelong habits. It required a composing of the mind and a soothing of what had always been a restless spirit. With fervor and a quiet urgency, Peter was working toward this final readiness.

In our conversations through the spring, Peter spoke of many things—ideals and disillusionment, the value of risk, the anguish and thrill of transitions—but the overriding theme was always the idea of becoming ready. Ready to live; ready to die. Ready to change directions when change was necessary.

Timeliness was everything. Opportunities were useful only to those who were prepared to seize them. Gifts were appreciated only by those whose minds were equipped to see their value. And nothing, not even death, is daunting to the person who is ready for it.

9

I'VE ALWAYS BEEN A FIRM BELIEVER in pushing my luck. For me, a phase of life is not complete until I've taken it as far as I can—or maybe just a little farther. Case in point: My brief career as a ski bum.

Let me tell you about the first time I ever did a double back flip off a ski jump, in my underwear.

This was in January of 1973—the year of the Green Truck. I was in Aspen. Aspen was anything but chichi in those days; it was an outpost of hippies and drifters, an old mining town with a great mountain and some pretty good bars. To pay for my lift tickets and cheeseburgers, I was doing odd jobs, things like stacking firewood or shoveling snow off of restaurant patios.

Then I heard about a new sport called freestyle exhibition skiing—or, more commonly, hotdogging. Seems that people would pay money to watch young lunatics do improbable things in the snow. Equipment makers would offer sponsorships to have daredevils show off what their then-state-of-the-art gear could do.

Getting paid for skiing! This beat the hell out of stacking firewood. I decided I would start competing.

I began with certain disadvantages. For example, my skis didn't match. What can I say? I lacked the funds to buy skis, so I'd bummed the intact halves of broken pairs. This gave me a certain tendency to turn left, but I learned to compensate. My boots were appalling, real ankle-breakers. My parka was an army-surplus job that leaked feathers.

Fortunately, at my first competition I didn't really need a parka. We performed practically naked—since the idea was to go rocketing off a ski jump and land in a swimming pool.

It was January, remember. But I was too young, too healthy, and no doubt too scared to be cold. I watched eight skiers go off before me. They all did flips. I studied them.

Here's a paradox: A braver person might have chickened out at that point. But I didn't have the nerve to admit that I didn't have the nerve. Once again, my insecurity egged me on. I had to prove that I could do it.

When my turn came, I barreled down the chute and leaped. I threw my head and shoulders back and hoped for the best. I saw sky; then the crowd; then snow. Then the same sequence over again. Then, thank God, after two full flips, I finally saw the swimming pool.

More by luck than by design, I made a perfect landing. My skis slapped the water, then held me afloat just briefly, like small pontoons. My heart was beating wildly as I settled into the pool.

By the way, I didn't win the competition.

I tell this story mainly as a way of illustrating something I said a while ago—about the importance of recognizing the difference between an acceptable, life-enhancing risk and one that's just plain dumb.

I realize that doing a double back flip off a ski jump could well be put into the latter category. But think about it. Eight people took the leap before I did. All came through okay. I'd gone to school on how they'd done it. And I'd be landing in water—a pretty forgiving substance.

True, I might have messed it up, flailed my skis, and looked like an idiot—but so what? You'll never accomplish anything if you're afraid to look bad trying.

Anyway, here it is, thirty years later. I'm so wasted and weak I can barely get up from a chair, let alone propel myself down a ski jump. Yet I still have the invigorating memory of that moment, I still recall the thrill of it. It was a risk that enriched my life.

Skiing, of course, offered all levels of risk, and some of them were, by any standard, foolish. I knew guys who, during competitions, would ski off cliffs—just go flying blind off of cornices thirty, forty, fifty feet high. What was beyond those mounds? Boulders? Trees? They had no idea. *That* was dumb.

Dumb or not, those moves were real crowd pleasers. So I started wondering if there were some sane way of working them into my repertoire. I thought about it, and came to a realization that's pretty obvious yet turns out to have all sorts of applications in life: *It's not the leap that's dangerous, it's the landing.*

The only reason a leap is scary is that a landing must inevitably follow. So why not plan that part first? Solve the problem of the landing, then work backward to the leap. If you think about it that way, the leap becomes the easy part. As I've said, no one gets hurt in the air.

So I started scouting cliffs. I noted where the hazards were and plotted my leaps to avoid them.

The onlookers didn't know this, of course. To them I was one more maniac. My cliff jumps still *appeared* to be headlong forays into unknown dangers. But I was not, in fact, a daredevil. Daredevils, sooner or later, get badly hurt, and I didn't have a death wish. I had a life wish. I still do. I was creating an illusion.

An illusion, by the way, that is useful in many avenues of life. Certainly in business, where the crazier, more volatile person usually has a negotiating edge. I devised a strategy I took straight from hotdog skiing: *Seem* reckless, but *be* prepared. Act crazy, but do your homework.

Not to digress, but I used to be a real wild man in meetings. I went out of my way to remind people that I was not entirely normal or predictable. I drummed on boardroom tables. I cracked jokes at entirely inappropriate moments. I threw tantrums now and then. I pissed off a lot of people. Others I only confused. But I always had a strategy. In every negotiation, every deal, I knew where I wanted to end up. Again, I'd planned the landing. That freed me up for all sorts of antics with the leap.

In all aspects of my life, then, I prided myself on being ready to confront the dangers up ahead. Whether it was trees in the snow, or the heart disease that killed my father, I believed I could prepare to face the hazards, and take decisive steps to overcome them.

Perhaps I was too cocky. Maybe I tempted fate, dared the gods to throw me some epic curveball.

Because cancer was something I never even thought about. Cancer? In my forties? Ridiculous. Outside the realm of probability. It didn't even run in my family.

In retrospect, I can't help wondering if there were danger signs I should have seen and didn't. Was I, like an American pedestrian in London, being vigilant by looking in exactly the wrong direction? Did I have some predisposition I was foolish not to recognize?

What if I'd run to the doctor on the first day I had the bellyache, instead of waiting for the feeling of wrongness to linger for a while? Would things have played out differently? Have I skied off a cliff I might have scouted better?

I'll never know, of course. And not knowing is one of those final frustrations that I've needed to become resigned to. Mortality doesn't limit us only in time. It limits us, as well, in what we can ever hope to understand.

◆ ◆ ◆

BEFORE I SAY GOOD-BYE to this part of my life, there's one more brief tale I want to set down. It's important to me to tell it, because, in my memory at least, it has a resonance that is almost biblical. It's about death in the midst of vibrant, over-flowing life; about horror and loss against a backdrop of the most sublime, majestic beauty.

During the winter that I skied my way across the West, I worked briefly on an avalanche demolition team in Sun Valley, Idaho. This was different from anything I'd ever done. I'd always skied for fun. When I took chances, it was in the name of competing or proving something to myself. Now I was skiing with a far more important purpose: to make the mountains safe for other people.

On patrol, we skied for miles and miles, looking for cornices, precipices, flumes where avalanches would likely start. When we found a potentially dangerous slide, we triggered it with sticks of dynamite that we carried on our belts. The avalanche would start to roll not far from where we stood. In the silence of the mountains it would build to a low whooshing roar, snapping trees, rolling house-sized boulders. A magnificent and humbling spectacle.

That was the preventive side of what we did. Then there was the rescue side. When unlucky or unwise skiers were caught in an avalanche, it was our job to save them, or to bring home the remains.

That's how I first saw death in the flesh, saw it not as a nasty rumor but a hard plain fact.

One afternoon the alarm bells started ringing. Four skiers were missing in a snowslide. One of them happened to be the wife of the man who owned the ski area. Her name was Mrs. Janz. We knew her slightly. She was a good skier and a nice woman. I tried to get my mind around the possibility that she was dead, broken and suffocated under tons of snow. It seemed impossible. She wasn't old. She wasn't sick. All she'd done was head out for a few hours of skiing. Could death be that abrupt, that random?

Our crew hurried to the site of the avalanche. The topography of it was terrifying.

Part of an overhang had broken off; part still remained and could go at any moment. We had to reconnoiter in the shadow of this remaining cornice. That's where the corpses were likeliest to be.

We started searching. Our technique was basic and macabre. We traced out a grid, then explored it step by step, poking through the snow with long fiberglass shafts. If we hit something solid, we stopped to dig it up. It was generally a rock or a clod of frozen earth.

But it could equally have been a person.

In the awareness of that, I realized for the first time in my life that death is not some abstract concept; it is a thing of weight and texture, a *specific* thing in each separate case. "Death" is just a word, a dim description; but the thing itself is a stunning event that happens to every living creature.

To Mrs. Janz. To me at some point. To everyone eventually. Basic, yes, but flabbergasting when you really grasp it—one of life's defining moments. Nothing looks exactly the same once you truly understand that you are not exempt from death.

I skied my portion of the grid. I poked my pole through the snow. I'm not sure which I feared more—that the overhang would crack, or that I'd be the one to find Mrs. Janz. I was nearly sickened at the thought of my hand encountering the frozen resistance of her flesh.

But, as the afternoon wore on, a different emotion insinuated itself along with the horror and the fear. It was awe.

The mountains were unspeakably beautiful, their sharp peaks golden above the tree line. The ravines, though treacherous, were magnificent rivers of snow. The air smelled of cold stone and pine; the sky was so blue it was lavender. The silence was broken only by the occasional low rumbling of some gigantic unseen motion.

Death was here too. Death was part of it. And I realized that it made no sense to say it was all perfect *except* for death. You couldn't subtract death from the equation. You either accepted the grandeur of the whole package, or you didn't.

Eventually, thank God, someone else found Mrs. Janz.

We put her body on a sled to bring her home, skiing through woods as the light was fading. Long purple shadows stretched across the snow. It was dark by the time we reached the lodge.

Along the way I had a peculiar thought. I thought about the odd phrase "gone to glory" that was used when someone died.

I forced myself to glance back at the corpse of Mrs. Janz, saw her body cradled against the dimming mountains and the trees. *Gone* to glory? She'd been in glory the whole time. I only hope she knew it.

10

THE RIGHT DECISION is the one you come to in your own sweet time. The good choice is the one you're truly ready to make.

As I've said, my generation has been fortunate in all kinds of ways. Unlike our parents' generation, we weren't pressured into marrying in our early twenties and starting families right away. Unlike the young people who've come along in less confident economic times, we didn't feel a desperate need to hurl ourselves too quickly into the hamster cage of commerce. We had the great luxury of picking our moments.

After my winter of ski bumming, and having passed the watershed age of twenty-one, I had the first inklings that maybe it was time for me to take some steps toward becoming a responsible adult. I'd paid myself back for my abbreviated childhood. I'd squeezed plenty of goofy, sexy fun into my extended adolescence. I was ready to move on.

I'd also met some people who'd been ski bums too long, and I didn't want to end up with a worldview as narrow as theirs—thinking about nothing but snow, moguls, and the newest model of Rossignols. I hankered to engage with the wider world, to try to figure out how it actually worked.

Not everything I learned was pretty. Some of it distresses me even now.

When the snow ran out in the spring of 1973, I found myself at Lake Tahoe, and fell into a job as a dealer in one of the casinos. This was great fun for a while: it was raucous and high energy, there was money to be made, human nature was revealed with every throw of the dice. Then I witnessed a really ugly incident. A woman colleague of mine was essentially ordered, if she wanted to keep her job, to have sex with a certain high-rolling customer.

I realized then that there was something fundamentally creepy about the morality of the gaming business. It wasn't just good, clean fun or people blowing off steam. The industry was built on an unwholesome confusion of money and power and sex and exploitation. I couldn't stick around after that. I still had at least some of my youthful idealism. Maybe I'd left behind the undergraduate dream of single-handedly changing the whole wide world, but I still believed that personal ethics mattered, and that individual choices made a difference.

So I packed up my stuff, drove back East, to Washington, D.C., and talked my way into a job with Common Cause, a nonpartisan, nonprofit group whose mandate was to restore faith in government by rooting out corruption and exposing antidemocratic practices.

I felt really good about working for Common Cause. So imagine my chagrin when I was fired—for daring to disagree with my superiors.

Getting fired from that job stung me twice. First, there was the sting of failure—and let me admit that I am highly allergic to that one. But there was also the sting of disillusionment. Common Cause was a bastion of free speech, after all; a guardian of Jeffersonian freedom! Yet the organization turned out to be as hierarchical and ego-driven as most others.

By now I was beginning to feel a little like Voltaire's Candide, the relentless young optimist who goes into every situation believing it's for the best and gets clobbered by life every time. The grown-up world was proving to be not such an easy place to navigate. But if Voltaire's wisdom applied, so, it seemed, did Woody Allen's: Success *is* 80 percent just showing up—if, that is, you show up willing to do almost anything, and to work your butt off at it.

It so happened that at the very meeting that got me fired from Common Cause, there was a quite renowned political consultant whose roster of clients included nearly half the Democrats in Congress. He liked that I'd spoken my mind. He thought what I'd said was pragmatic and reasonable. He came over as I was cleaning out my desk and suggested that we talk.

And so, just like that, I started running political campaigns.

The deal was this: I started my own company, which I named Partisan Artisan. The larger campaign-consulting companies would send me jobs that were too small for them to bother with. They'd take a cut of all fees, in return for which they'd teach me, on the fly, what the hell I was supposed to be doing.

I loved this. The learning curve was as steep as anything I'd ever skied!

My first campaign was a primary election for lieutenant governor of New York State, on behalf of a terrific young guy named Tony Olivieri (who, by coincidence, died of cancer in his thirties). When I took over, things looked hopeless. Come to think of it, I was pretty hopeless too! I knew nothing. I developed a tactic: When I was in a situation over my head, I looked down at my watch and said, *Oops, I'm late for a meeting!*

The "meeting" would be a frenzied phone call to one of my senior campaign adviser contacts in Washington, in which I'd brief him on what was going on and plead, *Now what do I do?*

He'd tell me. I'd do it. And before very long I became what I'd been pretending to be: the guy in charge. The guy who knew how to utilize party connections. How to organize rallies. How to work the media.

Did I feel like a bit of a fraud? Of course! Did I put ridiculous amounts of pressure on myself, trying to look confident? Absolutely. Was I afraid of falling on my face at every moment? You better believe it. But I loved what I was doing.

I've always felt that there are two elements of value in a job: the things we learn from the job itself, and the things the job teaches us about who we are and what we need.

Just as it took the challenges of Loomis to teach me that I loved to learn, it took the pressure-cooker atmosphere of political campaigning to teach me that I loved to work. As long, that is, as work was fun; as long as it had some content I enjoyed, rather than being just a grudging exchange of time for money.

I realized something basic then. If you work for fun, money will come. If you set out working for money alone, enjoyment is not likely to be part of the equation. If excitement isn't there at the start, why imagine it will come along later? A dreary job can only get drearier.

I learned, too, that as long as the adrenaline was flowing, my capacity for labor was almost boundless. I worked like a Trojan. I worked like a mule. At seven A.M. I'd be at a breakfast meeting with a ward boss or a minister or a rabbi who could deliver votes; at two A.M. I'd be drinking and strategizing with colleagues, reviewing the day.

Nineteen hours of concentrating; nineteen hours of running around. This perfectly fit my determination to live in double time. Was I tired? I must have been. Was this a healthy way to live? Not hardly. Did I notice? Absolutely not. Which might be the surest sign of pure type A behavior.

In fact, now that I recall the eager young man I was—my hair still longish but now neatly combed; my hippie duds traded in for wide ties and suits with big lapels—I suppose I could have been the type A poster boy. I had energy to burn, and I never stopped burning it.

I have no regrets about that; I was living large, dealing with real players. At the same time, I can't help wondering. . . . Did I shorten my life by assuming my life would be a short one? Was there an element of self-fulfilling prophecy in how hard I pushed myself?

One more thing I'll never know.

In any case, Tony Olivieri did not win the election. But we made it close. We made it exciting. And in the process, I caught the political bug. This would define the next decade of my life.

◆ ◆ ◆

JUST AS READINESS is the key to entering adulthood, it's crucial, as well, in facing one's mortality.

Earlier in these pages I talked about what I think of as the adolescence of my illness. I was like a hooked fish at that stage.

I knew I was in trouble but I'd had little time to ponder what was really going on. All I could think of to do was fight, and thrash, and wiggle. In doing so, I only wore myself out and caused myself more pain.

Eventually, I had to settle down. I had to arrive at a more candid understanding of my situation and my prospects. To put it simply, I had to start getting ready to die.

A transition like that doesn't happen overnight, but I roughly date the "adulthood" of my illness to the middle of 2001. By that time I'd had three major surgeries. My belly was a patchwork of scars; they arced and crisscrossed like the zippers on a high-tech parka. I'd had things removed, and things resewn, and the remaining pieces reconfigured. Back then I could still eat, but it was rarer and rarer that I was hungry.

I'd played out the string on radiation and chemo. I'd dealt with a number of doctors who'd run the gamut from the unforgivably callous to the amazingly kind. The bottom line, though, is that the doctors had failed. They were now reduced to trying to sound smart about how much time I probably had left.

Luckily for me, I had, by then, done most of the hard, strange work of separating my spirit from my physical self. I could almost accept the notion of my body as a beat-up old car that simply wasn't worth repairing anymore.

I say *almost* . . . because readiness isn't something that appears all at once. It's something you earn by increments, at the cost of much anxiety, and rage, and sadness.

This is one of the most difficult things I have to talk about in this book. Because I really want my story to be of comfort—but not at the sacrifice of honesty. And the truth is that getting ready to die is tough and painful—more so, I believe, than the merely physical torments that define a bad disease.

When people write about death and dying, they tend to use terms like *resignation* and *acceptance*. I suppose those catchwords provide a useful shorthand, but they're also potentially misleading. Nothing is, in fact, that simple.

Resignation isn't a single emotion—it's a dance of a hundred emotions that sometimes rise to philosophical detachment, then descend again to the most desperate, childish clinging. Acceptance is not a onetime goal, like the crossing of some imaginary finish line; it's a process of a thousand starts and stops, a multitude of tentative but failed approaches toward peace of mind.

Back in 2001, I sometimes had calm days, grateful days, days when I told myself I was becoming resigned. Then, at night, I'd wake up from terrifying dreams, sweating, breathless, frightened. What sort of resignation was that?

Most of the time I didn't feel well. I'd started dropping weight. I continued losing strength. These dispiriting developments served, at least, to further my readiness. . . . But then I'd have a day or two of feeling strangely good, of having energy and appetite. And I'd start believing that a miracle was happening, that the disease was mysteriously receding, that my body was confounding science and battling back. This was readiness?

Or I'd have moments of deep peace, times when I felt a profound satisfaction that my life's work had been accomplished, that I'd earned my release and could start letting go. . . . Then I'd be visited by sorrowful and maddening thoughts of all the things I'd miss by dying: I wouldn't see my kids graduate from high school and college. I wouldn't walk my daughter down the aisle. I wouldn't have the leisurely adventure of growing old with my wife.

If there was such a thing as resignation or acceptance that was powerful enough to be an antidote to those sorrows, I knew I hadn't found it yet.

As I've said, though, I don't mind working hard if I believe a job to be of value. And as my attitude toward my illness started to mature, I came to understand that getting ready for the end, facing it with style and awareness, was the most important task I still had left to do.

11

WHAT I NEEDED after that first failed primary campaign was two days of sleep, and a week on a beach somewhere. What I got instead was an immediate offer to work on the election bid of New York gubernatorial candidate Hugh Carey.

The opportunity was too good to pass up. So, in a pattern that was already becoming familiar, I traded rest and balance for excitement and ambition. Why not? I was healthy and young. I was also, as usual, broke. I took the job at once.

If I'd been in the frying pan with Tony Olivieri, I was right on the coals with Carey. This was the big time, a New York governor's race. Moreover, Carey had a real shot at winning. The pressure was ridiculous. Nobody talked, they screamed. They didn't negotiate, they threatened. Every day was a potential calamity, every move either a coup or a colossal blunder.

If I had the time, I could tell a lot of war stories from that campaign. I learned some nifty tricks: making rallies seem bigger than they were; bamboozling the media into reporting on support that wasn't there. I saw how future favors were bartered for present help. Rather than go into detail, I'll just pass along the old observation that successful politicians are like hot dogs—if you like them, it's better not to watch them being made.

In any case, Carey did win the election, and while I didn't exactly ride his coattails into state government, I did, some months later, become a part of his administration. The way this happened says much, I think, about the shifting prospects of my generation, and also about the person I was at that stage of my life.

It was 1975. The economy was in the tank. Remember stagflation? Suddenly nothing seemed to be working very well. Companies forgot how to make money. Jobs grew scarce. This was nerve-wracking. It forced people my age to think, maybe for the first time in their lives, about security. Maybe the gravy train *wouldn't* last forever. Maybe opportunities ran out, after all. Maybe it was time to hunker down and latch on to something.

But what? The fact that I chose state government reveals a truth that at the time I hid even from myself, but that now, with the bracing candor that comes with being close to death, I can readily admit: I had a lot of bluster but very little confidence.

I acted brash and cocky, but secretly I feared that everyone knew more than I did. I asserted myself not out of real strength, but because I was afraid I'd otherwise be overlooked, that I would disappear.

There's no surprise in a truly brave person acting brave; it's when the erstwhile coward rises to the occasion that we feel pride in our humanity. Similarly, it's no great accomplishment for a genuinely confident person to seem confident. But I had to work at it every time. I had to suck up fear over and over again. (This, by the way, is a trait I seem to share with many of the most successful people I have met in business.)

Anyway, with due respect to civil servants, I chose government work in part because I felt it was an arena that wasn't exactly chock-full of world-beaters, so I'd have a chance of standing out. And, false modesty aside, that's pretty much what happened.

I joined the Carey administration as a special assistant to the commissioner of agriculture. Within a year, I was working full time for the governor himself—full time meaning fourteen hours a day. I was either overseeing or actually running a dozen different agencies. Helicopters ferried me back and forth between Albany and Manhattan. I had my very own unmarked state trooper car in which to tool around on official business. I was twenty-five years old.

Those were heady times to be in government. When economic times are good, the private sector views the public sector as a drag on progress and a nuisance. But when the economy is lousy, the gung ho capitalists come running to the government for help. We saw plenty of that in the middle seventies.

We also had the unique situation of our greatest metropolis teetering on the brink of financial collapse. New York City was about to default on its bonds and go bankrupt, remember? I worked with the Municipal Assistance Corporation to help fashion the bailout.

I also proved, beyond a doubt, that I was not an advertising genius.

The crisis facing New York City was not only a fiscal one; it was also a crisis of morale. The city's image was at a low ebb. Tourism was down. People were depressed. New York State decided to fund an ad campaign to restore the city's glamour and appeal.

The job went to the firm of Wells, Rich, and Greene, and I was at the meeting where the formidable Mary Wells first unveiled her brainchild. As usual, I was impatient, jumpy. Time was being wasted on stroking and formalities. There were too many suits around, too much ceremony. I looked for an opening to blow things open—to use irreverence to get back to the real. The opening came when Mary Wells stood up and explained the centerpiece of the proposal.

With my characteristic subtlety and tact, I chimed in that it was the dumbest thing I'd ever heard in my entire life.

Fortunately, I was voted down, and the "I ♥ NY" campaign went on to be the most successful and widely imitated PR blitz in history. Belatedly, I jumped on the bandwagon and helped fashion some of the tactics that made it work.

What it comes down to is that I was awfully young, and no doubt I made some dumb mistakes, but I was really in the thick of things, and it was as exciting as hell.

Let me tell one story that for me encapsulates the excitement of those times, the sense of privilege. It's not about politics. Inevitably, I guess, it's about music.

One night, Frank Sinatra came to Albany. I can't even recall if he was there for a concert, or to receive an award, or what. But, sometime around midnight, he showed up at the governor's mansion. I happened to be there, hanging with some of the Carey kids.

Hugh Carey was a true Irishman—loved to drink, loved to sing. He didn't sing well, but hey, he didn't have to—he was the governor. After several rounds of beers, he started singing Irish songs.

Then he seemed to remember that there was a grand piano in the drawing room. "Hey, Pete," he said, "why not play 'My Way' for Frank?"

Me? Play for Frank Sinatra? The notion was utterly terrifying. "Um, maybe I'll just go to the pantry and fetch more beers."

"Great idea, Pete. Fetch some beers and then we'll sit around the piano."

There was no way to say no, so I started playing. And, to my everlasting amazement, Frank Sinatra—Frank Sinatra!—started singing along. Thank God I remembered the chords. It didn't go badly. Loosening up, I segued into "Witchcraft," "Fly Me to the Moon," "That's Life." Beer kept appearing. Sinatra kept singing, his famous vocal cords just a few feet from my ears. Together—together!—Sinatra and I improvised a medley that just went on and on. When I floated up from the piano bench it was well into the wee hours.

I didn't know it then, of course, but I was almost at the precise midpoint of my life.

Half my days and nights were behind me; half lay up ahead. Moment by moment, I was both filling up and using up my destiny, amassing memories I would cherish forever.

Sitting in a governor's mansion, making music with Frank Sinatra . . . I could hardly believe how fortunate I was. I have trouble believing it even now.

◆ ◆ ◆

REFLECTING ON MY GOOD FORTUNE in life is part of what I do to bolster my readiness to leave this life. True, I haven't had the full span of allotted years, yet I have the quiet satisfaction of believing that there's nothing I have missed. Reminding myself of that is a pleasant job, and not a difficult one, since the evidence of my great good luck is all around me.

I'm fortunate enough to live in a comfortable home, in a setting I find very beautiful. Everything about the place has meaning for me: the pictures on the walls, the mementos on my desk, even the dog toys and chewed-up tennis balls on the floor. I love it all.

The house is saturated with the life of my family. I find old Legos between the cushions of the sofa. Lost jigsaw puzzle pieces and single mittens sometimes come rolling out of cupboards. I feel a crazy attachment to these small domestic details, an attachment that is even sweeter for the recognition that it will soon be broken.

A couple of years ago I planted some new trees between the house and our little pond. Ash and maple and cottonwood. I already knew that I was dying, that I'd be gone while the trees were still in their fragile infancy. Was I groping after some version of immortality? Was I trying to fulfill the old Chinese proverb that the current generation plants trees so that future generations may enjoy the shade? I have no idea; I didn't need to stick a label on it. I planted trees because it pleased me to plant trees. Now I see them straining against their stakes and wires, trying to bend into the shapes they were meant to have, each one determined to be unique. I love that.

I love it, too, that my house is full of noise.

Some visitors have been surprised at this, even rattled. They've felt that a house with a sick person in it should be a quiet place, a hospital zone. My own feeling is that there'll be plenty of time for silence, thank you very much. In the meantime I take a tremendous joy in clamor.

I love it when Jeff is listening to hip-hop while Chris is blasting the television and Kate is screaming above the din to a girlfriend on the phone. If Laura happens to be yelling out chore assignments for dinner, so much the better. This family noise is the music that's beyond music. This is vitality. This is life.

And of course it's my kids, way more than anything else, that remind me every minute how incredibly lucky I have been on this earth.

My children know I love them. If I'm sure of anything, I'm sure of that. But I wonder if they realize that even the smallest details of their lives have been unspeakably precious to me.

A scrawled homework assignment left out on the kitchen counter. A baseball cap sitting crumpled in a chair. A silly rambling joke told at the dinner table. Can my kids possibly understand how much those little things have enriched their old man's life?

Some people, I think, ask way too much of Heaven. They want it perfect. Perfect, unchanging, and safe. They're looking for a payback for things that weren't great down here, an escape from uncertainty, from the ups and downs and noisy messiness of life. I see it very differently.

I don't begin to have a vision of what's on the Other Side, but what I hope from it is far more modest.

I'm not looking for an upgrade of my life on earth, because I frankly can't imagine what an upgrade would be like. I feel that if I'm half as fortunate in the Hereafter as I have been right here, then that'll be as much as I, or anyone, deserve.

12

LIKE EVERYBODY ELSE who ever went to Sunday school, I was taught as a kid that money is the root of all evil.

I neither believed nor disbelieved this, any more than I believed or disbelieved any of the other axioms that we were taught at Sunday school. They were grown-up sayings; they didn't sink in very deep at the time. They were notions to tuck away and draw conclusions about in later life.

Well, my conclusion is this: Money is not the root of all evil. But maybe the *lack* of money is.

Worrying about money is dreadful. Being too preoccupied

with money is crass. Being hard up for funds leads to shortsighted decisions, and can tempt good people to do dumb, bad things.

I realized this on the evening that a Saudi prince tried to buy my political help with a plain white envelope stuffed with cash.

This was in 1980. I was still working in state government, and loving it. I made a very modest salary, but I felt I was doing something of value. Part of my work was in economic development. I helped create jobs. I helped reinvigorate blighted areas.

In the course of my duties, I met a member of the Saudi royal family who was thinking of locating several businesses in New York State—an investment of a couple hundred million dollars that would bring in thousands of new jobs.

I liked the prince a great deal. He was smart, polished— and he drove a hard bargain. We met half a dozen times, and negotiated with gusto. He was always looking for tax breaks and concessions; I was trying to cut the best deal for the state. Finally, I thought we had an agreement. We jumped into his limo and went off to celebrate with a dinner at Tavern on the Green, in Central Park.

But on the way to the restaurant, the prince blindsided me with demands for one more round of concessions. I told him I couldn't do it; it was beyond my authority. He responded that if I could just get him a one-on-one meeting with the governor, he was sure that we could close the deal.

And then, across the limo's leather seat, he slid an envelope bulging with what seemed to be a wad of money.

I was so flabbergasted that I didn't immediately realize what was going on. No one had ever tried to bribe me before. For a moment I stared at this perfectly ordinary envelope as though I simply couldn't figure out what it was. Then I got embarrassed. Then angry. I was terribly disappointed in the prince. I'd started thinking of him as a friend.

Without a word, I got out of the car at the next red light.

Then, standing somewhat dizzily on the sidewalk, I realized that a taxi back to my office would cost me around $4.50. That was a lot of money!

Well, guess what? The Saudi prince turned out not to be a prince at all, or a Saudi either, but an undercover FBI agent, part of the soon-to-be-revealed ABSCAM sting that resulted in the prosecution of several high-level politicians. Hugh Carey and a few of his aides, myself included, had been targets of the sting. So were numerous state and federal officials from throughout the Northeast.

For me, this episode left a really sour taste, for a couple different reasons. First, if one branch of our government felt the need to use such sneaky tactics to entrap members of another branch of government, then I wasn't sure I wanted to keep working in government. The whole thing was a little too KGB for my comfort.

I had more personal qualms as well. I can honestly say that I was not remotely tempted to accept that bribe. I followed my gut reflex, which was to walk away. Then again, I was twenty-nine, and single; I thought about fun and satisfaction, not money, and my modest salary was adequate for my needs.

But what if I was forty-five and still a civil servant? What if I had a wife and three kids? What if my kids were strapped for tuition or if someone I loved had gotten sick and needed expensive treatment? What if someone tried to bribe me then? Could I be absolutely certain I wouldn't be tempted? I didn't think I'd let myself down . . . but could I really be sure?

It's funny, in a way—our society warns us about the temptations of wealth and power, about the slender chances of a rich man getting into Heaven. But poverty has its pitfalls, too. Too little dough can erode a person's ethics and values just as easily as too much.

In any case, shortly after the attempted bribe—in one of those radical and abrupt direction changes that have defined my life—I decided I was leaving government and going private sector. I'd come to the quite conscious conclusion that I needed to spend the next ten to fifteen years making money.

And this may sound crazy, but it's true—I needed to do so, in part, to safeguard my honesty. I hoped that, on the off chance that I had a normal life span, I might return to public service someday. If that happened, I wanted to make sure that self-interest would not be the driving part of the equation.

In the meantime, I had a really strange hurdle to overcome. I had to launder my résumé of the "taint" of government work. Which is really perverse, if you think about it. While employed by New York State, I oversaw billions of dollars and was involved in the destinies of millions of people. Yet so great is our society's bias against the public sector that I still had to prove to the world I could be "businesslike." So I applied to Harvard Business School.

The B school turned out to be both the worst and the best thing for my confidence. By the time I went there I was almost thirty; my classmates were twenty-three and twenty-four. I felt that 95 percent of them were smarter than I was. One hundred percent of them were more technologically savvy. They all had fancy handheld calculators that spat out precision to five decimal places. I still used—no kidding—a slide rule!

Suddenly I was part of an older generation. I used different tools and had a slightly different outlook from that of the people around me. How can I put it? I was way out-whizzed by a whole new breed of whiz kids.

The first year's workload was ridiculous, and everybody else seemed to power through it with less sweat than me. I toiled away in constant fear of flunking out. Failure may not have been an option, but it was a strong possibility nevertheless.

Having made it to the second year, however, I started seeing things from a more complex perspective. Okay, my classmates were analytically brilliant and precise. But precise in the name of what? Of figuring out the unit costs of widgets? What purpose would be served by their impressive calculations?

I became increasingly mistrustful of their sterile precision. I started suspecting that their obsession with detail was a way of masking cluelessness about the bigger picture. When we were bailing out New York City, we ran our numbers with a slide rule. If a slide rule was accurate enough for rescuing the greatest city in the world, wasn't it accurate enough for estimating the profits of some company?

I also began to realize something else about my fellow MBA candidates. It's a sweeping generalization, but I stand by it. In the main, they weren't excited about the *content* of their eventual careers—the actual work they'd do—but only the rewards. They didn't want to create. They didn't want to take chances. They wanted to find a safe track that offered money and prestige; they would gladly settle for a bland, predictable "success."

Bottom line: They were extremely bright people who would never really *do* anything, would never add much to society, would leave no legacy behind. I found this terribly sad, in the way that wasted potential is always sad.

I began to understand—at last!—where my own advantage lay. Certainly not in brains. Certainly not in social polish or family connections. My edge had to do with something more visceral, more basic: I had passion. Passion, and some measure, at least, of creativity.

I didn't want a safe niche; I wanted to make something that wasn't there before. I didn't want to manage; I wanted to invent.

If I crashed and burned, so be it. But there had to be some big dream worth pursuing, and there had to be joy and excitement in the challenge of pursuing it.

My classmates could analyze, but I, thank God, could rhapsodize. In business as in life, that's a far more precious thing.

◆◆◆

TO AN EXTENT that surprises me, I rhapsodize even now.

Illness has shrunk my world in both space and time. Waning strength has limited my options. Most of what we ordinarily call pleasure is history for me.

Yet I take pleasure from each and every day. True, the pleasure often coexists with pain. True, the pleasure often takes the form of recollection. But so what? It's pleasure nonetheless, and I savor it.

There's a solemn game I'll bet that all of us have played at one time or another. The game consists of trying to decide at what point life would no longer be worth living.

We hear about a friend going through chemo, losing her strength, losing her hair, and we secretly wonder if we ourselves would find it worthwhile to press on.

Or we read about some unlucky person who is paralyzed in an accident, and we can't help thinking that death would have been a less cruel outcome.

Or we see loved ones stricken by chronic pain, or Alzheimer's, or any of the many misfortunes that can turn a life into a tormented shadow of itself, and we wonder if there could possibly be a point in continuing.

Well, one of the things I've learned from having cancer is that it's always worth it to continue. Death will come when it's ready to; the bad stuff will end. You can count on that—and I don't think it's morbid to consider it a comfort.

But in the meantime there continues to be good stuff, too.

Small pleasures loom large. As with anything in short supply, their value rises with their rarity. A favorite two-minute song can offer all the satisfaction of a symphony. There's rapture in watching a dog chase a tennis ball. Sometimes a breeze from the west carries a pine smell down from the mountains.

Redemption. There's another word I've never really thought about till lately, another one for which I don't pretend to have an airtight definition. But if there is such a thing as redemption, it doesn't happen only once, or all at once.

I think we're redeemed at every moment we find something good among the bad, something joyful in the sorrow, something to continue being grateful for.

I sometimes think about a scene from a favorite old movie, *My Dinner with Andre,* one of the most improbable movies ever made. It's basically a quiet Socratic dialogue overheard on film.

Andre is a romantic, an aesthete, a perfectionist. He tells his friend Wally that, for him, a great day has to be sublime in every detail. There has to be a perfect meal at a perfect table overlooking a perfect sunset. One flaw anywhere and the whole experience is spoiled.

Wally is just the opposite. He asks very little of life. He's thrilled with whatever scraps of pleasure the world throws his way. A good day for him is when he wakes up in the morning, finds a cup of coffee left over from the day before, and discovers that no cockroach has crawled into it and died.

Well, when I was young and healthy, pumped up with the brightness of my prospects, I wanted to be Andre. Demand the best. Insist on perfection.

But later in life, humbled by sickness and the prospect of mortality, I've come to understand that Wally, all along, was really the wiser person, and certainly the happier one. He had the great gift of being pleasantly surprised, of seeing small delights as large victories.

A person of Andre's temperament would have a really tough time getting ready to die. He'd grumble at every bodily insult, mourn every vanished possibility, see every lost pleasure as a personal affront. A person like Wally, on the other hand, is already so much closer to acceptance and to peace.

Thank God I'm becoming more and more like Wally.

IF ONE ADVANCES CONFIDENTLY IN THE DIRECTION
OF HIS DREAMS, AND ENDEAVORS TO LIVE THE LIFE
WHICH HE HAS IMAGINED, HE WILL MEET WITH A
SUCCESS UNEXPECTED IN COMMON HOURS.

—Thoreau, *Walden*

⋄ ⋄ ⋄

AS THE WORLD moved toward summer—the prime of the year—Peter's story pressed forward, toward the joyful but foreshortened prime of his life.

Through June and July, we sometimes had the pleasure of chatting outdoors in the baking warmth. Locusts buzzed. The afternoons smelled of fresh-mown grass. Occasionally Peter would interrupt himself to listen to the insects and to savor the air. Then he'd resume his tales of what he'd done, and what he'd learned, in the years when his strength and drive were at their peak.

His eyes lit up when he recalled those shockingly recent times. His mouth often broadened into a grin still full of mischief. Even so, there was a vivid, painful contrast between the person telling those stories and the person who had lived them.

Peter, as a healthy man, had been a whirlwind of energy, had thrown off sparks in all directions. His boldness was propped up by a personal philosophy, but its true source was something more visceral: a physical vigor and sheer animal zest that now were gone forever. I realized, sadly, that there were sides of Peter I might hear about but would never know firsthand.

By June, Peter had already outlived the doctors' estimates of his longevity, and the mere act of sustaining life now claimed much of his power. He was often tired. Fatigue frustrated and embarrassed him and sometimes made him irritable. Irritability, in turn, led him to become more private. He began withdrawing from many of the people he'd been close to—especially the hale companions of his most active years.

As Peter saw it, old friends could not help pitying him, and he could not abide their pity. Most of all, he grew weary of saying good-bye. "Each of my friends," he told me, "has one good-bye to say. I have hundreds. It's exhausting."

Peter's friends missed him, missed him even before he'd passed away. His new privacy was a radical reversal of his life-long sociability; it took people by surprise, left a gap in their affections.

As a new and different sort of friend to Peter—a friend for his dying—I stayed within the orbit of his shrinking world. And so a tenuous but heartfelt brotherhood sprang up among some of Peter's old friends and myself—among men who, even weeks before, had never met. It was as if we formed a cabal whose purpose was to keep Peter alive—alive not in his flesh but in our hearts—by sharing what we knew of him.

I could report on Peter now—his courage, his frankness, his undiminished curiosity. But in the swapping of Peter stories, I got far more than I gave—because old friends could flesh out the part of Peter's life that I would never see; they could tell me of Peter in his tireless and undaunted prime.

One friend told me: "I've never seen a person pack more life into a day. And I've never known anyone with such an appetite for putting himself at risk. One time we were mountain-biking down a glacier. Peter took off straight down the fall line.

No chance of stopping. I was sure he'd kill himself. Sure enough, he hit a rock and went ass-over-teakettle. He got up with blood streaming from his forehead and an absolutely ecstatic smile on his face—like he'd beaten the fear, he'd faced it down."

Then there was the notorious "Barton curve," as a former colleague explained it. "No one could wing it like Peter. One time, in the early days at Liberty, he was making a big presentation to investors. He got up, drew a set of x and y coordinates, and put in a beautiful, sweeping growth curve. Only, he was so excited, he didn't write in any units on the graph. Was the time line months or years? Was the money millions or billions? Did Peter even have the numbers, or was he bluffing—just drawing a map of his own optimism? No one ever knew."

Another friend spoke of Peter's legendary impatience. "The man just couldn't sit in traffic. I don't mean he didn't like to—I mean he couldn't. I remember one time I was sitting in a horrendous traffic jam on I-25. Suddenly I see a flash of red go by on the median. It's Peter in his Ferrari. I feel this mix of admiration and resentment—the way you always feel toward someone who gets away with things you yourself don't have the nerve to do. A little while later I see Peter stopped, getting a ticket. I can't help thinking: Serves him right! . . . But damned if he doesn't pass me again a few minutes later, still driving on the median."

Irreverent; outrageous; boyish. These are the words that come up again and again when old friends speak of Peter. "As in

Peter Pan," says one. "He never quite grew up. Kids understood that, and loved him for it. A touch-football game, a water fight—all the kids wanted to be on Peter's team. My son used to say, 'Boy, if I had an older brother, I'd want it to be him. He's just so cool!'"

My own contribution to the cabal of Peter's friends was essentially this: I was able to report that Peter had, in fact, grown up at last. He hadn't shed his basic playfulness or forsworn his lifelong optimism. But his formerly scattered energies had finally come together and were focused on the ripest goal, the only one that matters in the end: achieving peace of mind.

Through that summer, a season that Peter never thought he'd live to see, he taught me that just as there is a prime of life, there is a prime, too, in the process of approaching death.

If life's prime corresponds to the period of greatest physical power, then the prime of dying is defined by strength of spirit. In this other prime, Peter mustered an unflinching awareness and maintained it in the face of awful pain, and battled to keep it whole even as concentration became an ever-greater challenge. He made an array of choices as bold as any he'd ever made before: He chose gratitude over disappointment, curiosity over complaint, hope over despair.

Somehow, he transformed fear into a bracing suspense; he reshaped death itself, so that it was no longer a gaping terror, but just one more of life's intriguing twists.

13

By the time I got my MBA, I was thirty-one years old and really in a hurry. I didn't think I'd live past forty-five, remember, and in grown-up terms I hadn't yet done anything. I had no savings and no career. I wasn't married, and my long and rollicking bachelorhood was starting to feel tedious and stale.

I was beginning to acknowledge something that, deep down, I'd already felt for quite some time: that I was put on earth to be a husband and a father. Whatever else I might accomplish would be in support of that. Raising a happy, loving family was the main event.

But I was also an intensely practical fellow, the sort who sat down and did the math—who thought about the landing before I took the leap—and I didn't want to start a family unless I was sure I could afford one. So I had to get cracking.

I launched into the process of applying for jobs. Not surprisingly, my approach was rather different from that taken by most of my classmates. Most Harvard MBAs apply to the biggest firms in the most established industries—investment banking, consulting—and, like racehorses at an auction, they sell themselves to the highest bidder in terms of starting salary.

I began by setting my own starting salary: zero.

That's right, I wanted no money at all for the first ninety days. Then, following this free test-drive, my employer could fire me with no further obligation. But I could also fire him. I didn't have the time to wallow in a situation that was going nowhere.

Working for free, of course, was part of a larger strategy. I had other demands that were far more important to me than a number on a paycheck.

I would only work for someone I thought was wildly smart.

I would only work directly for the head of a company. That, I felt, was the only way to learn fast and advance fast.

I would only work in an up-and-coming industry. (This, by the way, is something that still amazes me about so many of my classmates. These people could analyze anything, yet most of them followed the herd into mature industries whose greatest days were behind them. Why didn't they take half an hour to analyze where the real action, the real growth, would be?)

As a matter of personal preference and quality of life, I would only work in Boston, San Francisco, or Denver.

Well, with all those conditions I was clearly limiting my options. But I did my homework, and I came up with a list of possible employers. I started with a personal Who's Who of 231 names and sent each of them a letter. Amazingly, 123 CEOs responded. For various reasons, that group was gradually whittled down to three possibilities in Denver. There was a hippy tea company and two cable-television outfits.

The tea people didn't really want me, and one of the cable companies was already top-heavy with MBAs. That left a dinky little outfit called TCI, which was headed by a seat-of-the-pants, feet-on-the-desk visionary named John Malone. From our very first conversation I realized that Malone was the guy I wanted to work for. He thought huge. He was informal, original, and totally audacious.

If this was a business book, I'd write a long chapter about why cable was such a fabulous opportunity in 1982. But basically it comes down to this: The industry was essentially a government-subsidized monopoly, financed with huge tax breaks. It was young and fragmented—there was big money to be made in the process of consolidation. The capper was that most of the small operators didn't see the big picture, didn't realize the value of what they had, and didn't have the nerve or vision to put the pieces together. John Malone did.

So, after Malone agreed to hire me, I went back east, threw all my stuff into a big yellow Ryder truck, and drove it out to Denver. Everything was rush-rush-rush—exactly the way I loved it. I didn't even take the time to find a place to live, just moved into a TCI company apartment that was little better than a Quonset hut.

I'd barely unpacked before Malone had me out on the road, buying up everything in sight. Back then, every town seemed to have its own cable provider—mom-and-pop companies with ten thousand or twenty thousand subscribers; astonishingly, in the early 1980s, TCI was acquiring outfits like that at the rate of one every four days! The cash flow from one deal financed the next. Some of the time we barely knew what we were buying. But we were in a classic race to get big fast.

Fast, of course, had always been a favorite word of mine. Now I began to see that *big* could also be a lot of fun. You could do cool stuff with *big*. In some ways, you could change the world. I was having a great time.

Then one day, about a month into my employment, Malone called me into his office. Rather sheepishly, he told me that our ninety-day trial was off. He had to put me on the payroll—the accountants had told him it was a liability thing. We agreed on a salary of thirty-two thousand dollars a year. As a starting wage for a Harvard MBA, this was pretty chintzy. Still, I was so busy, and so excited about what I was doing, that I forgot to ask for a raise for three years!

At the same time, though, whenever anybody left TCI, I made a point of offering to buy the stock they'd acquired as an employee. This hints at a paradox that I really can't explain very well, but that I think a lot of people will understand. On the one hand, I really didn't care about money. Thirty grand a year or sixty grand a year—so what, as long as I was getting by and doing something I liked. On the other hand, once I realized the growth potential of the cable business, I started thinking, for the first time in my life, that it would be pretty satisfying to accumulate some real wealth.

Dollar by dollar, money was a grimy reality. But there was something pleasingly abstract about a fortune. It wasn't a pile of cash this high or that high. It was an experience—a peak adrenaline rush not so different from playing the Apollo Theater or flipping backwards off a ski jump in my underwear. It was extreme. It called for creativity and the testing of one's nerve. It was a goal that existed at the outer limits of our generation's possibilities.

History had given us rock 'n' roll, and hippie vans, and the luxury of time to figure out our true ambitions. Now I was being presented with an opportunity that, conveniently enough, had materialized just at the moment I was ready to seize it. I began to see that helping to build an enterprise, and making some real dough in the process, was more than just a practical affair. It was an adventure suited perfectly to the next stage of my life. I went for it.

✦ ✦ ✦

GOING FOR IT, of course, is the way I've almost always done things. It's so much a part of my temperament that it's almost beyond the reach of conscious choice.

Going for it is the way I dealt initially with my disease.

My response to cancer was nothing if not active. I studied up. I formed a strategy. Then, I attacked. With surgery; with chemo; with every damn therapy I had access to.

It's not a coincidence that so many of the words and metaphors people use in speaking about cancer sound military. A person battles the disease. Or mounts a campaign against it. The fact is, I saw my illness as an intimate little war, with my own ravaged abdomen as the battleground. Maybe that was good for my "fighting spirit," but in terms of accepting my situation and becoming resigned to the fact that my disease was terminal, I see now that I probably made things harder for myself.

From the patient's point of view, cancer seems like a deeply personal affront. Like any other insult, it makes you angry. But if you think about it, cancer really isn't personal at all. It isn't an "enemy." It has no bad intention, any more than a fungus on a tree has bad intention. A tumor may be malignant, but it isn't malicious; it just has an agenda that doesn't fit in with ours. We're the ones who define the relationship as a "battle"; the disease is only doing what its chemistry is telling it to do.

Still, when we are cured of something, we like to say we "beat" it. We congratulate ourselves on our immune system and our courage. But what happens when we don't beat a disease? Does that mean we've lost, been defeated, failed? That our courage has been lacking? In addition to the pain of sickness and the wistfulness of watching our time running out, do we also have to take on the shame and humiliation of feeling that we've let ourselves down somehow, that we've come up short in the most crucial fight of our lives?

Maybe these are only words, but the feelings that go with them are real. And, as part of my getting ready to die, I had to go through those feelings and find a way to relieve them of their sting.

Gradually, I had to stop thinking of my illness as a fight that I would either win or lose, and begin to understand it as a mysterious process that was bound to run its course. My disease and I were not opponents, we were more like unwilling room-mates forced to live in the same tight quarters of my body. Maybe it wasn't a happy arrangement, but it wasn't warfare either. It was an uneasy coexistence that would continue for a certain length of time, and I had to get on terms with it. I had to accept the annoying truth that I was no longer in sole control.

In the course of doing that, I realized something useful: that acceptance doesn't mean the same thing as giving up.

The distinction is subtle; the language isn't perfect; but I can tell you from personal experience that I'm not just playing with semantics here.

Giving up is when you're in a contest and you acknowledge that you've lost. Acceptance is when you graduate to a different way of looking at the situation. You make peace with the obvious fact that the outcome is no reflection on your character; you no longer see it in terms of winning or losing. Somehow you leave those opposites behind. It's a big relief.

There's another way, too—a more positive way—in which my tendency to go for it has defined my attitude toward my disease. This has more specifically to do with facing death. It might sound weird or morbid, but the fact is I'm excited about dying. I wouldn't mind putting it off another twenty or thirty years—but that's a different issue.

Given that my death is inevitable, I'm genuinely interested in what it will be like. I'm curious as hell. I'm not just passively sliding toward the moment, I'm imagining it all the time. I've always prided myself on having a zest for each new phase of life. Why should that zest evaporate when the next phase is dying?

I'm not saying that fear isn't part of the equation. Fear of death is natural. I'm sure it's hardwired into us. Which is a good thing—it keeps us from leaning too far over the edge of the cliff or canoeing too close to the waterfall.

I've been learning that as death grows imminent, the fear of it no longer serves a purpose. And so it falls away. Not entirely. Not all at once. But it grows milder, gentler. The panic drains out of it.

Then again, there's fear at every one of life's big transitions. Fear goes with the territory. And I see that as an opportunity. Fear makes us study ourselves, forces us to admit our soft spots, to see where we are vulnerable. In the end, we can't undo that vulnerability; we can only accept it, and crawl forward in the face of it. That, I've had to learn, is part of being human.

I've said before that I have no dogma or even any confident guesses about what's on the Other Side. But I have an ever-strengthening hunch that there must be something other than oblivion. I have too many thoughts left, too much curiosity, too much love still stockpiled for family and for friends. I can't believe it all just stops.

I want to find out.

I hope that, when the moment comes, I'll have the courage not to cower, but to meet death in a hearty, open-armed embrace. I hope I'll have the nerve to cross over without a qualm, with as light a spirit as if I were heading out on one more cross-country jaunt, blasting the radio in one more moving van, singing along at the top of my lungs.

14

TCI LAUNCHED me on my improbable journey to becoming a wealthy man and a person of some influence in the media business. But it did something far more important for me as well. TCI is where I met my wife. I first saw Laura Perry at a company Christmas party in 1982.

For two decades now, I have stood by the weak fib that she was smitten with me at once. Fortunately, I've never fooled anybody with this feeble lie; and of course just the opposite was true. I met Laura and *my* life changed. Or maybe it's more accurate to say that a change I was ready for now had the perfect reason to happen.

Laura was beautiful. She was smart. She was strong in body and in will. She had humor and lightness coupled with a rock-solid character. She was not a person to be trifled with.

And she was justifiably wary of me. I was a hyper executive, nine years her senior, very full of myself, on the road a lot. I had a lousy record with relationships. Sure, I'd been dumped a couple of times, but usually I'd been the one who decided when something began and when it ended. My so-called love life had been equal parts passion and convenience. Mea culpa—I'd thought of women largely as a form of recreation.

Relationships had been one of those aspects of life in which I made things harder for myself, was too feisty for my own good. I'd waffled on commitment. I'd sometimes been unkind simply by inattention, being too wrapped up in other things. I don't think I'd ever truly let someone into my life.

I was also saddled with the odd and macho notion that a man needed different sorts of women at different ages. In his twenties—so I'd thought—he needed blithe playmates, footloose companions who were always up for a road trip or a three-day hike. But in his thirties, a man started looking for a woman to make babies with, and so his priorities became quite different; now he looked for sanity, seriousness, strength of character, and values. In his forties, he needed someone sexy and adventurous enough to let him feel he was still virile, still exciting. And in his fifties, he hoped for someone who was still beautiful and beckoning and, in addition, unfailingly dignified and charming enough to buoy up his fragile ego in any social situation.

What I was too dumb to realize, of course, was that if you were lucky enough to meet the right woman, she was all those things and more—and the two of you evolved *together*. When I met Laura I finally started understanding that.

And thank God I did. When I think—with a guilt I can't quite conquer—of the emotional rigors that Laura has gone through because of my illness, I am amazed at how much ground we've covered, how much we've faced together.

It boggles my mind that my new thrilling lover of just a few short years ago is now the unimaginably courageous partner who will see me through my death. From Laura I have finally learned to trust without reservation. She loved me when I was strong. She loves me in my weakness. I still find this miraculous.

Back at the start, I courted her as I had never courted anyone. I was determined not to blow it. Previously, if there were difficulties, rough patches in a relationship, I walked. Now we worked things out. Previously, I did things my own way, by reflex. Now I was willing to pause, to see the wisdom in Laura's way. It was crucially important to me to get this right, because I had the absolute conviction that if Laura and I started a family, we would stay together forever.

I do not believe in divorce where there are children involved. I realize I'm a bit reactionary on this subject, and I don't care. I think that, especially in a culture where premarital experimentation is not only accepted but encouraged, divorcing is selfish and wrong. The kids end up scarred; anyone who feels otherwise is kidding himself.

Anyway, Laura and I dated for around six months, then started living together. I was experiencing something I'd never felt before—delight and excitement and regard that just kept building, way past the infatuation stage. I was closing in on thirty-five and had finally found the love of my life.

At length, I proposed marriage—in a hot-air balloon, thousands of feet above the highest of the Rocky Mountains. (That's partly why we went ballooning this Easter, to relive that stunning moment.) My head was literally in the clouds.

I tried to keep the proposal a surprise. But it wasn't so easy smuggling a bottle of champagne, a pair of crystal flutes, and an engagement ring into the basket. Laura noticed that I was acting a little strange. Of course I was. I was just about bursting with my secret.

I popped the champagne at around sixteen thousand feet. In the thin air, the cork blasted out like a rocket. I poured the wine. Laura and I linked arms, as in the King Arthur stories. Then I dropped the ring into Laura's glass. I can still picture it twinkling amid the bubbles. I told her that if she wouldn't marry me I would have to leave the room. . . .

Boy am I glad I rented that balloon! I have savored this memory five thousand times. I savor it still. You've got to go over the top for romance now and then. It's a way of making life exalted. It sweeps you out of the everyday, but also reminds you how precious the everyday is. I mean, when that balloon came down, this amazing woman and I would go *home* together. . . .

◆ ◆ ◆

TALK ABOUT LIVING in double-time: While I was courting Laura, my emotional life was more intense than it had ever been, but I was also working as hard as I had ever worked, traveling the country doing deals for TCI.

It was grueling, but finally it paid off. Near the end of the eighties, I reached the only financial milestone that has ever seemed significant to me: I banked enough money to feel that I could raise a family in a situation of comfort and security.

It happened, not surprisingly, in a slightly crazy way.

I said a while ago that, given the torrid pace of TCI's acquisitions, we had to learn an awful lot, awfully fast, or we wouldn't really know what we were buying. Well, the deal that assured my family's future was one in which we had to do more than just research a company; we had to appraise the potential of an entire industry that was just then coming into being.

In 1986, it was something new under the sun: home shopping. Home shopping on television. Who ever heard of such a thing?

We got into the home shopping business by way of a Minneapolis-based mail-order company called COMB—a low-tech operation that essentially sold closeout hardware through a catalog. COMB's founder, Irwin Jacobs, thought it might be spiffy to hawk his goods over the airwaves. He contacted us to suggest a partnership.

John Malone and I flew to Minnesota to look the company over. Jacobs, along with one of COMB's senior executives, picked us up in the exec's Rolls-Royce. Compared with the car, however, the rest of the business was a letdown. The warehouse was funky, the computers antiquated.

Still, Jacobs was on to a great idea. Greater than he realized. I grandly told him that if he turned us loose to transform COMB into something we'd call CVN—Cable Value Network— and to take it national, we would get him ten million subscribers within a year of when we launched. He laughed. The executive laughed. To stop them laughing, I told them I'd bet a Rolls on it. We shook hands.

By the agreed-upon date, we were in seventeen million homes. I still have that executive's car.

The launch of CVN was an exercise in frenzy. I ran all over, trying to get cable system operators to carry the network. Since home shopping was so new, there was no model for what kind of deal to offer. Everything was a guess, an improvisation; this was business as boogie-woogie, and I loved it.

Disaster shadowed our every success. Sales boomed, but our computers couldn't handle the volume. We ran out of stuff to sell. We literally had people dashing down to KMart and Target to get more merchandise to offer.

It was a messy beginning, but CVN really took off. Within two years it was a billion-dollar business with forty-six hundred employees. But I'm a start-up guy by temperament, and by then I was tired of running it. The only way to make a graceful exit was to merge the company with another recent start-up called QVC.

At this point I could finally sit still long enough to consider my stock options. I saw what they were worth—three million bucks, a million and a half after taxes!—and cashed them in at once.

Now, some people might say that a million and a half dollars is not a lot of dough, but to me it was that most elusive amount: enough.

Enough so that I was confident my wife and kids would be secure.

Enough so that everyone would have a home and tuitions would be paid.

Enough so that if I dropped dead tomorrow, everyone would be okay. I was over the hump. I could do right as a father.

I was thirty-eight when that money came to me. More money has come, as money does; it takes on a momentum of its own. But the rest has been Monopoly dough, just a way of keeping score. Only that first windfall felt real. It put my life on a different, far less pressured footing. I had so much pressure to let go of—I sometimes feel like I've been exhaling for a dozen years.

◆ ◆ ◆

DURING THOSE DOZEN YEARS, Laura and I have savored a life full of love and fun and one of the deepest satisfactions that people can have—the making of great kids. I sometimes think there must be an afterlife, if for no other reason than so my gratitude for these gifts can continue. Of all the things I can't imagine just suddenly stopping, my thankfulness and wonder for the life I've had is near the top of the list.

That life is ending. I know that. I'm reminded of it with every mysterious and wandering pain in my belly, every time a nurse comes to the house to dress a wound or re-tape an IV connection.

I'm part of a hospice program now. My care is what's known as palliative. The first premise is that I am surely dying. There's no illusion of a cure; I'm to be made as comfortable as possible. This is a mercy, and I'm extremely grateful to the kind and, above all, realistic people who look after me. At the same time, there's something galling about their attention. What their attention means is that I'm very sick and I'm not going to get better.

Honestly, I still find this a truly difficult idea to grasp.

We've all been sick many times in our lives. We've always recovered. Why not this time? Why not now? Illness has always been a temporary setback, an excuse to linger in bed and sip tea. Nothing prepares us for that one illness that doesn't go away.

Lately, the hospice people are urging me to start taking medication for the pain. There's quite a range of drugs to choose from, quite a number of ways to circumvent the whole digestive tract. There are patches you can wear, "lollipops" that release their medication straight into the capillaries of the mouth. There's a dispenser with a button you can push to shoot morphine right into the bloodstream.

Before too much longer, I guess, I'll have to start the drugs, but for now I'm just saying no.

I'm a control guy—I'm well aware of that. I've had to make my peace with losing control of many, many things; the last realm where I still have dominion is my mind. I'm not yet willing to surrender on that front, because there are still some issues between now and the end that worry me. I'm afraid of getting wiggy and undignified. I don't want my family to see me that way. I don't want to linger on as a doped-up zombie. I really hope I'll be spared that.

Besides, even without drugs, there's something hallucinatory, something surreal, about the prospect of dying. Every now and then I am visited by images of my life—images as vivid and persuasive as anything psychedelic—but it's my life *without me in it.* This is a hard thing to explain. What comes to me is not a thought. It's not about implications, or even emotions. It's purely visual. It's fleeting. It's a tease, like a trailer for a movie.

Here's my desk chair, but I'm not sitting in it.

There's my piano, but the keys remain untouched.

There's the family dinner table, but with one fewer plate and knife and fork.

When I see these images, it's as if I'm already gone. It's like I'm looking back, not just from a great distance, but from somewhere altogether different. It's a little creepy, sure, but it's also strangely comforting. Things remain in place without me. Life does, in fact, go on.

And, to a degree at least, I can control the images. If they become disturbing, I can blink, and swallow, and yank my mind back to a more normal mode. If I don't like the pictures, I can make them go away. I'm not sure I'll be able to do that once I start the pain meds. I'm afraid that drugs will shift the balance— that the images will control me, rather than vice versa. This concerns me. I don't want my last thoughts to be like one of those annoying, obsessive fever-dreams from which you can't wake up.

One of the things I pray for, wishing on my stars, is that it doesn't come to that.

15

I WON'T PRETEND that I'm thrilled to be dying in my prime. But the situation does have a few advantages.

Most people's lives, I think, follow the shape of a bell curve. In youth, the graph gradually ascends, as people gain in strength and education and, most important, a sense of who they really are. Then there comes a glorious plateau—that part of adulthood when prowess and joy and confidence are at their height. The plateau, in turn, is followed by a gentle decline, a gradual letting go of vitality and influence, either a mellow or a bitter slide toward the end of life.

Well, my graph doesn't look like that.

On the ascending side, I more or less follow the usual pattern. But somewhere along the prime-of-life plateau, cancer comes into the equation, and my curve becomes more like the track of a ball rolling off a table.

This is not a complaint. Because what it means is that I am never far away from my happiest days, the days when I was healthiest, and most assured, and living the life I had dreamed of someday having.

My memories have not had time to take on a sepia tinge; in fact, my recollections seem far too recent and immediate to quite be memories at all. I think of my prime as something that lasted until yesterday. I picture its details in wild, living color, and hope to do so until the day I die.

A person's prime, I guess, is an approximate notion; it doesn't start at one particular moment. But if I were to pick a point at which my life reached its richest, and most fulfilled, and most complete stage, I know exactly what it would be: the moment I became a father.

It was 1987. We were still living in Minneapolis. I remember Laura's pregnancy as a crescendo of incredible suspense. It proceeded step by exquisite step—from her first intuition that she'd conceived, to the confirmation that a new life had started developing inside her, to the first amazing sonogram, that curled and blurry image of our daughter.

To me, Laura got more and more beautiful as the months

wore on. I won't presume to guess what a pregnant woman thinks or feels or goes through, but I will say that, viewed from the outside, it seemed that she had glimpsed the final secret of the universe and come away with an almost otherworldly serenity.

She was doing the most important work there is. Despite the physical discomforts, this gave her a focus and a calm and a certainty that a man could only admire, and maybe even envy a little.

We decided early that I would be there at the birth and would participate in whatever ways I could. I would not have missed it for anything in the world.

I held Laura's hand as we counted the seconds between contractions. I encouraged her and stroked her forehead as she labored.

When the baby first presented, I grew woozy with excitement and terror. And when the newborn Katherine McCord Barton was free and breathing on her own, I cried with joy. With trembling hands, through tears, I cut the umbilical cord.

And I was intensely aware that I was in the presence of a miracle.

I've always gone back and forth on the God thing. I still do, even now. But at the birth of each of my children I have felt the undeniable presence of some version of a supreme being.

Maybe it's just that I love my kids so much that I need to believe the world they will inhabit is a benign one and has meaning. Maybe I need to trust that there's a someone—a sort of ultimate playground monitor—who will ensure that my kids are treated fairly by the universe, who won't allow them to be bullied or hurt.

In any case, with the beginning of a family there comes the start of family traditions, family rituals.

I've said earlier in these pages that for many years now I've been in the habit of wishing on a star each night. That habit began on the night our first child was born.

I needed to worship, to give thanks. I needed to pray for her well-being. Call me pagan—standing alone under a cold, crisp November sky and mumbling to the stars struck me as the most natural and honest way to do those things.

As our family has grown with the births of Jeff and Chris, my prayers have gotten longer, taken on more texture. I give myself a lot of leeway when I wish on stars. I ramble. I scatter my wishes with no great discipline. Ultimately, though, all the wishes and all the rambling comes down to one unchanging plea for the health and safety and happiness of my family. What else matters next to that?

Other traditions were also born along with Kate. It became a sacred custom that I would be there at each birth—and each was as thrilling as the one before. The suspense remained sublime. And, to my unending fascination, I saw that each of my children was born with a fully formed personality that has never changed. From her first breath, Kate has been feisty and fiery and determined. Jeffrey Spencer Barton emerged from the womb as the same mellow, observant, and amiably private boy he is today. Christopher Perry Barton was all sweetness and humor from the first moment he saw daylight, cuddling and cooing. Where did those different personalities come from? That's another miracle.

It became a ritual that I would sever the umbilicus, doing my bit to welcome my children into life, to help start them on their way. I became so unashamedly superstitious about this that I even wore the same shirt every time. My birthing shirt.

I still have it. As a garment, it's nothing special—heavy cotton, pink and white stripes, a little frayed around the collar—the kind of shirt you throw on with a pair of jeans. But it's been spattered with tears, sweat, and the blood of my family. It's one of my most prized possessions.

◆ ◆ ◆

WE CUT THE CORD at the start of each life. In a different way, we cut the cord at the end. We have to say good-bye.

I find, by now, that I have very little problem saying good-bye to my own life. I've lived it. I've savored it. There's no way I feel cheated. Would I prefer to grow old? Sure. But it's not my choice to make. I'm okay with that.

The thought of saying good-bye to my children, however, is agony. It's the one thing I just can't seem to get reconciled to. I'm sorry to say this, but I think it's a sadness without an antidote.

I've groped after comforting thoughts on this matter. I've told myself that it's the natural order: Parents see children through the start of their lives; children see parents through the end.

I know that, but it doesn't seem to help. I feel that, in regard to my kids' lives, I am exiting far too early. Maybe I'd still
feel that way if I lived to be eighty. But the fact is, I'm going now,
when my daughter and sons are children. I can't shake the feeling
that I'm letting them down; for all my progress toward acceptance, this one aspect of dying makes me sick at heart.

Selfishly, too, I mourn all that I will miss of their lives.
When I think of the challenges and discoveries that my children
have before them, I am full of boundless curiosity and giddy
hope. I'm thrilled at the prospect of everything they'll learn and
accomplish. That I won't be here to see their destinies unfold fills
me with helplessness and frustration.

This is the anguish of a parent. I can't pretty it up. It hurts
like hell.

My only solace is to remind myself that there has also
been great joy—joy that has compensated me ten times over for
the grief I'm feeling now.

Nothing raises the stakes in life like having kids. Suddenly,
the future matters. Emotions take on an amazing resonance. Love
bounces off the family walls and multiplies. Everything you do
with your kids lives on in their memories as well as yours; everything's more valid because it's shared.

Let me tell you about the best hour of the best day I've
had since getting sick.

It was just a few months ago. It was becoming pretty clear
that my days for gallivanting were just about over, so Laura and
I decided to join the whole family—kids, siblings, nieces and

nephews, parents—for a cruise in the Caribbean. There were twenty-one of us in all.

Physically, I did very badly on the boat. My GI tract was in the process of shutting down; the motion was torture. But so what? I wasn't there for my health. I was there to do something wonderful with the people I love. This was nearly the last time there would be a fabulous payoff for disobeying the docs and being a really lousy patient—I wasn't about to miss an opportunity like that!

The best day was in Jamaica. It so happened that an old media industry friend of mine—Chris Blackwell, who introduced Bob Marley to the world—owns a small resort there. It's called GoldenEye, originally Ian Fleming's home, and is all but impossible to get into. At Chris's invitation, we were welcomed to have lunch and spend the afternoon.

Now, if I came from an old-money background, maybe I'd be awfully blasé about this. But in fact my family hadn't had a lot of opportunities to hang out in places like GoldenEye, and I took a great deal of pride and pleasure in being able to host them there.

Who knows—maybe I still have things to prove. If that's the case, I do not apologize. Bottom line: I was in a spectacular place with the most important people in my life, and I was in my glory.

Which brings me to the sweetest hour of all.

I took my daughter Kate out on a jet ski. I wasn't supposed to get wet, let alone go pounding through the surf. I didn't care in the least. These were unspeakably precious moments; my spirit wasn't about to sacrifice them to the problems of my body.

We zipped and bounced along. Kate held on to my back; her cheek was against my shoulder. It was like she was a little girl again, and I a young and healthy and protecting father.

We explored a bunch of little coves around the resort. The water was a hundred shades of blue and green; sunlight glinted off it so brightly that it almost hurt. Rays scudded by; tiny fish went skittering across the surface. Everything amazed us; we just pointed at things and giggled.

And we talked about how great life is. How lucky we were to be living it. As a family and as ourselves.

I choke up when I recall this story. But not because I'm sad. Because there's more joy in the recollection than I can hold. There was a lifetime's worth of pleasure in that single day—an intensity and a completeness that strike me as a great deal more important than the mere question of how many years a life contains.

That excursion on the water taught me that each moment is a life, that life is renewed every time we're walloped by beauty, every time we're shaken up by gratitude and love.

I have nothing to complain about. I feel like I toured much of Heaven in that single afternoon.

16

In 1988, with the home-shopping business up and running, and with Kate in tow, we moved back to Denver. The following year, Jeff was born; in 1992, Chris came along—and with those happy events, our family reached its final form, and my own life was filled up to the brim.

By coincidence—maybe—that completeness happened just after I turned forty. And it tickles me that, for all my detours and dubious decisions, for all my false starts and occasional screwups, my life's most robust and chock-full stage was beginning right on schedule, almost to the day!

Again, this was great good luck. The world had cut me plenty of slack. I don't think I'd done one single thing on the usual timetable. I'd raced through school, then dawdled on the road to a career. I'd stalled and stalled on marriage, then embraced fatherhood quite soon.

At any given moment, I was either ahead of, or behind, the beat. Yet by the time I turned forty, my life was right where it should be. I firmly believe there was a kind of generational inevitability about this. We lived as we chose, and more often than we probably deserved, things worked out. Amen.

By further coincidence, I was just forty when my career evolved into its ripest phase. That phase dates from 1991—the year that Liberty Media was founded.

Whole books have been written about Liberty and the genius behind it, John Malone. For now I'd just like to say a few very basic things about the company.

Liberty became a famously complicated enterprise—Wall Street analysts had the damnedest time understanding it—but the central idea was simple enough to put into a single sentence: We wanted to forge partnerships between the people who owned cable systems and the people who provided programming.

These partnerships, we felt, would be of benefit to everyone. Cable operators needed varied and targeted content that wasn't available on free TV. Programmers needed start-up capital, and a guarantee that there would be outlets for their programs. Liberty made money—a lot of money, as it turned out—

by facilitating deals between the people with the ideas and the people with the wires.

Often we invested in the resulting businesses. Thus, we ended up with significant equity stakes in CNN, the Discovery Channel, Black Entertainment Television, Home Shopping Network, the Family Channel, MacNeil/Lehrer Productions, STARZ!/Encore, and Court TV, to name just a few.

Through the nineties, the money snowballed. But the thing I'm proudest of about Liberty is only indirectly connected to its financial success. What I'm proudest of is that the company became a sort of temple for entrepreneurs. People trusted us enough to bring us their ideas. If we believed in their smarts and their passion, we funded them and left them alone.

I was privileged to be, among other things, a gatekeeper in this process. I listened to hundreds of pitches—everything from home-team-only sports to a crazy idea called MTV. I helped to shape dreams—to move notions into the realm of the possible. I worked at the intersection of the creative and the practical, and it was an amazingly exciting place to be.

I love entrepreneurs. I am in awe of people who can come up with a fresh concept and by sheer will make it a reality. There's nothing I respect more than that. Let's face it: 99 percent of people in business just move preexisting pieces around the board. Entrepreneurs create. If they are very good at what they do, and if they have some luck thrown in, they may leave behind something that will continue after they're gone. Believe me, I think a lot about such things these days.

I learned a lot from working with creators.

I learned what an exhilarating leap it is to put one's faith in another person's instincts. I learned the subtle art of helping without interfering.

Most managers counsel prudence and caution. At Liberty, we urged just the opposite. We wanted our entrepreneurs to be bold almost to the point of recklessness. I had a personal credo that I also advised others to follow: Don't ask permission, just beg forgiveness. If you're going to make a mistake, make it with your foot on the accelerator. If you drive with one foot on the brake, you're not for us.

God, this was fun!

People worked their butts off at Liberty. Because the other remarkable thing about the company was its extraordinary leanness. In the early nineties, we were a multibillion-dollar concern with sixteen employees! This was absolutely unheard of. We had no bureaucracy and no dead weight. Every person in the company wore several hats and accepted huge responsibility. Other outfits of similar resources were like armies with too many generals and a mass of privates trying to look busy. We were a commando unit.

Have I made it clear that I loved my work? Then I hope it will be equally clear that I love my family a whole lot more. That's why, from the first day our kids were born, I made myself a solemn pledge: I would not, for any price, allow my career to turn me into an absentee father.

With due respect to my own dad, I did not want to become one of those harried executives who made it to one Little

League game per season. I didn't want to miss precious moments of my kids' growing up—the first lost tooth, the school play—by being off on business trips. I didn't want my kids to have to get to know me all over again after I'd been gone for weeks.

I made myself a promise that, whatever else was going on, I'd be home every evening by six. With only the rarest exceptions, I held to that pledge for the rest of my working life.

I didn't do business dinners. I didn't do business cocktails. I drove our corporate pilots crazy. If I had a meeting in New York, I'd schedule it for nine A.M. This meant leaving Denver at four in the morning.

But it also meant I could be home in time to hear about my kids' days, maybe to throw a ball or help them with their homework. I hope this was good for my children; I know it was good for me.

Not only was, but *is*. I savor these family moments in the present tense. They are with me all the time. I smile about them in private.

As I've said, I guess the good part of dying in my prime is that my fullest days are still so recent, still so fresh in my mind. I think of dinner table conversations still waiting to be finished, funny stories that are bound to have their sequels.

In a peculiar way, it's like everything now happens at once for me. Past, present, what's left of my future—they're all right there in front of me at every moment. Nothing is in front and nothing is in back. As in a painting with the perspective flattened out, everything is right there, available. I'm very glad of this. It makes the moments amazingly rich.

Many lives grow thin and stale before they end. I feel grateful that my life will not have time to taper very much. I want to go out with a full heart, and five things in my mind at once, and a desk cluttered with projects I fully intend to get to, maybe the day after tomorrow.

◆◆◆

ADRENALINE and accomplishment at work. Love and noise and peace at home.

Sports, music, food, and wine. Lovemaking and deal making. Program launches and long walks in the mountains. . . .

Life is gloriously complicated. But if life is so wonderfully complex, why would anyone imagine that death is simple? Death is as much of a roller coaster as life itself. How could it be otherwise, given that death is part of life?

In the thoughts I've set down about the prospect of my dying, I've been somewhat inconsistent. I'm well aware of that.

At moments I've managed to write with an almost Hindu sort of calm, and just a little while later I've been frustrated and angry. Here I admit that I've got nothing to complain about, and there I go right on complaining.

In one passage I can suggest that I'm grateful for all the

things I've learned from having cancer; in another passage I'll rail at the doctors, and suggest that my getting cancer is the dumbest and most unfair thing that ever happened.

I make no apology for these inconsistencies. I'd rather be honest than consistent. Consistent isn't how it feels.

I don't have an agenda; I'm not positing a system here. Frankly, it strikes me as sort of silly to suggest that there are four steps or twelve steps or a hundred steps to getting ready to die. Who's counting? I'm just trying to give a candid report of what I've experienced and continue to experience, to map the progress toward my own little death. I don't pretend that it's been tidy.

Maybe, toward the very end, simplicity reigns at last. Maybe the contradictions resolve. Maybe the emotional static subsides, and all you hear is one fantastic, settled chord.

I don't know, I'm not there yet. It would be beautiful if it came to that; I'd love to hear that chord, and tell you what it sounds like. But who knows if I'll be able to report back by then.

In the meantime, I'm still trying to track the ups and downs.

Lately it's become more difficult, because of the pain medications I've had to start taking. This is a fine irony for a baby boomer: I can now have all the drugs I want; they're legally delivered to my house; I'm *urged* to take them in ever greater quantities—and of course I don't want them at all.

It's not that I'm stoic about the pain. I hate the pain. The pain is wearing me down as much as the disease.

It's that the drugs present a pretty beastly trade-off. I can have less pain at the cost of less awareness. Less discomfort if I'm willing to begin to disappear.

Unless I'm kidding myself, I'm still lucid most of the time. But I can no longer take my clarity for granted. I have to *choose* it. I have to work for it.

It's become almost an athletic kind of thing. I have to gear up, warm up, focus, do without the pain meds for a while. And I know that every mental workout will be followed by a deep fatigue. That's the price to be paid for each bout of concentration. I have to keep believing that the thoughts are worth the price.

I'm young enough that I can still remember being a little kid who didn't want to go to bed. I remember feeling the total, played-out tiredness that kids go through at the end of the day. I remember feeling cranky, irritable—knowing that I'd be happier asleep, that sleep would be a great relief.

But still, stubbornly, probably against my own best interests, I fought to stay awake. I was afraid of missing something wonderful.

I'm still afraid of missing something wonderful.

FOR US BELIEVING PHYSICISTS, THE DISTINCTION
BETWEEN PAST, PRESENT, AND FUTURE IS ONLY A
STUBBORNLY PERSISTENT ILLUSION.

—Einstein

"WANNA SHOOT some pool?" says Peter.

At first I think he's kidding.

It's been a couple weeks since I've seen him. He's spent much of that time going back and forth to the hospital—inpatient, outpatient, emergency room—dealing with a series of setbacks, the kind of inexorably linked and escalating discouragements that track the progress of terminal disease.

He's had a new tube inserted, to get around a blockage in his gut. The procedure led to an infection, with a fever that spiked to 105 degrees. To manage the crash from the fever, the doctors pumped him full of fluids; he put on an astonishing twenty pounds of water weight.

Finally, the infection was controlled; the fever gradually subsided, as did the grotesque swelling occasioned by the excess hydration—at which point it was found that the tube did not function as was hoped. It failed to open up a passageway now choked with cancer. It didn't relieve the pain. Peter went home a notch more beat up than he'd been before.

Disappointment after disappointment. Crisis after crisis. This is Peter's reality now.

It's no exaggeration to say he's at the point where any little thing might kill him. A chilly day could rob him of the core heat he needs to stay alive. A hot day could dehydrate him, starve his brain to the point of coma. Something could shift in his abdomen and strangle an artery, causing it to burst. He has become so fragile that he could die of a coughing fit; he could die of the sniffles.

But meanwhile, he wants to shoot pool.

So we go down to the Barton playroom, through a stairwell wallpapered in family photographs. The family skiing. Peter canoeing. The family arrayed around a vintage motorcycle.

Mixed in with the vacation pictures are more formal photos of Peter with the famous and the powerful. There's a sly lack of hierarchy in the arrangement of the images. Bill Clinton and Al Gore smile next to a shot of the kids dressed up for Halloween. Robert Redford and Ted Turner beam importantly, while in the next frame the Bartons are tossing snowballs in their parkas.

Peter's house is big—but not so much so that the life of his family doesn't fill it up entirely. Down in the playroom, Kate is doing homework while simultaneously giggling into the telephone. Chris and Jeff are watching videos in the mini-theater. Peter closes the soundproof door and pops a CD into the stereo. Paul Simon starts wailing "Gone at Last" while I rack up a game of eight ball.

Not surprisingly, Peter's a pretty good pool shooter, determined and precise. Even encumbered by his knapsack, he handily outplays me.

But after two games, he's exhausted.

Healthy people grow tired by degrees, but there's nothing

incremental in how fatigue comes on for Peter. For him, weariness is an ambush, a collapse. It's abrupt and overwhelming, and it offends him deeply. Suddenly wobbly, he shakes his head as he puts aside his cue. "This is ridiculous," he says. "I'm hitting the wall already. Let's sit awhile."

The kids have gone upstairs. We plop down on a sofa in what is now a quiet room. Peter puts his feet up on an ottoman. I notice that his ankles are still puffy from the fluid imbalance, and that he is wearing white elastic socks.

Unembarrassed, he sees me looking. "Yeah," he quips, "I've taken to dressing like my grandmother."

He lets his head loll back a moment and reaches in a pocket for a narcotic lollipop.

The pain medicines have now become a fact of life for Peter, an accessory both merciful and despised. He seems to see the drugs as a capitulation, a giving in; he started taking them only when he was finally persuaded that the pain itself had become more draining and more of an obstacle to clarity than even narcotics would be. Even so, he's very grudging with the medication; he doses himself like a stingy bartender. Two licks of the lollipop and it's returned to his pocket.

I ask if it helps.

Peter pauses to think the question over. He still analyzes things, still strives to be exact. "It doesn't stop the pain," he says. "It's almost more a spatial thing. It seems to move the pain farther away. . . . Bear with me. I need a little rest."

He closes his eyes. In the stillness I hear his IV pump; it runs in humming pulses broken up by clicks.

In two minutes—no more—Peter blinks himself awake. His eyes find their focus, and he flashes me the warm, unguarded smile that is one of the privileges of our intimacy. "I'm back," he says.

I smile in return. But I'm troubled. It's become clear to me that time itself is beginning to break down for Peter.

Duration, for him, is no longer quite the same as it is for most of us; he sees time not in terms of days or hours but in episodes of energy, bursts of attention. This highly personal clock will inevitably isolate him. Healthy people more or less agree on how time is paced, how a day is divided. That consensus is an aspect of what links us; time is part of our community.

But eternity is a timeless place, and the dying seem to prepare for it by dissolving time beforehand.

Over our next several conversations—the last that we would have—Peter revealed how profoundly his sense of time was changing. He'd always been a thoroughly logical man; he remained so even now. But the central premise of his logic had been altered. It was no longer based on sequence—cause and effect unfolding over time. Rather, his logic now organized itself around patterns and recurrences.

Things happened—and happened again in the act of their remembering. Old feelings were new in the moment they were recalled. Recollected sights were no less real than the images before his eyes. Things lost long ago were found once more. Broken things and fractured emotions were whole again. Nothing had faded.

During the course of his final weeks, Peter grew calm. No doubt, this was partly due to sheer exhaustion, and to the benign effects of medication. But seeing him, talking with him, I became firmly convinced that there was another cause as well. Peter grew calm because, for him, there was no longer any tension between the past, the present, and the future. His entire life was available, compressed, in every passing instant.

As time lost its dominion over him, Peter came ever closer to reaching the goal of all religion and all philosophy: seeing things in their completeness, and accepting that everything that is, must be.

17

SOMETIME AROUND THE END of 1996, I threw myself
a party.

It was a very odd sort of party, in that it didn't happen at
any particular place or time, and no one but Laura and I realized it was happening at all. But it was a celebration nonetheless,
complete with champagne, and a giddy break from the usual
routines, and even the counter-current of melancholy that often
goes with parties.

The occasion was not a birthday or an anniversary. It was
the fact that I had now outlived my father.

This was a huge milestone for me, as well as a genuine surprise. I was forty-five and a half years old and my heart hadn't yet given out. All those hours on the treadmill, all those years of saying no to the butter and the Brie had paid off.

Having expected a radically short life, and having pushed myself accordingly, I now felt like a gambler playing with house money. No matter what bet I made next, I was ahead of the game. I'd *won*. I could elbow in at any table. There was a freedom and a gratitude in this that almost made me dizzy. I was determined to make the most of it.

On April Fools' Day of 1997, at a breakfast meeting with John Malone, I resigned as president of Liberty. I was a few days shy of my forty-sixth birthday.

From everyone's perspective but my own, this decision seemed wildly abrupt and unexpected. But in fact it was part of a long-considered plan. It was never my intention to keep that— or any—job forever. I only like a job when I'm still learning, when I really don't know what I'm doing, when I can feel the thrill of performing without a safety net. After six years at Liberty, I was doing things by rote. Why? To make more money I didn't really need or even want? To prove to myself that I was still a player?

The reasons to continue seemed woefully inadequate. And truthfully, the cable industry was not nearly as much fun as it had once been. Success had made it dull. Its vast size had rendered it conservative. Inevitably, huge and sluggish organizations now controlled it.

Besides, I was ready for a new adventure. You could call it a midlife crisis—except that I was way past midlife, and besides, I had a "crisis" every decade or so. Now, again, I felt a hankering for one of those extreme and exhilarating direction changes that have defined my path and kept me juiced.

My possibilities were nothing short of mouthwatering. False modesty aside, now that I was in my prime I had the resources and the connections so that whatever I did I could reasonably expect to do it at the highest level.

From my days in state government I had retained an unwavering belief in the value of public service. Now, because of relationships I'd forged within the Democratic party, I had reason to hope that I might at some point be tapped for an ambassadorship.

I still loved media, and thought my knowledge of that field might be helpful in the nonprofit arena. I explored the notion of running National Public Radio.

The entrepreneurial side of business still excited me, and the Internet, in 1997, looked more than a little like cable TV had looked in 1982. I spoke with the boards of Yahoo, AOL, and Microsoft about creating a billion-dollar incubator for promising e-commerce companies.

Yes, I was thinking big. And loving it. My life was still tracing out my generation's happy arc. Next stop: elder statesman.

But here's something that's slightly embarrassing to admit. I've acknowledged before that true confidence did not come naturally to me; insecurity has been a constant companion and a constant goad. And in 1997, even as I was fantasizing a great next phase, I was secretly afraid that, without my job title, I would quickly be forgotten, pushed aside. Peter who? What's he done lately? I honestly worried that people would no longer take my calls.

Maybe I'm paranoid. Or maybe the business world really is that fickle. Either way, the fear was real enough. And now that I think of it, maybe that's partly why the writing of this book has become so important to me. It would be comforting to feel I've done something that can't be so easily erased.

In any event, the dilemma of my next big plan soon became moot. Blindsided by cancer, I watched my grand schemes go out the window. Yearning for health, working for survival, became my major occupation.

I'm wistful, of course, about the things I might have accomplished and didn't. Success—make no mistake—is the ultimate baby boomer drug, and, in my middle forties, I craved another dose. But if illness put the kibosh on my exploits in the wider world, there was a compensating good that came of this: it focused my attention on things closer to home, on more intimate arenas where, I hoped, I could still make a difference.

So, for instance, I volunteered to teach a class in the business school of the University of Denver. I wanted to preach the gospel of entrepreneurship. I wanted at least some small number of MBAs to understand that their real mission lay far beyond mere number crunching or consulting.

I started the Privacy Foundation, a nonprofit resource dedicated to helping people protect themselves from unwarranted snooping, especially through the Internet, by government and commercial interests.

But the thing I feel best about is that, freed from the demands of conventional "work," I had the great privilege of getting involved, in a really hands-on way, in my kids' education.

I'm not talking about the schoolroom here. I'm talking about exposure to the real world.

One day my kids had some friends over. I eavesdropped as they were having the what-does-your-dad-do conversation. When it was Jeff and Chris's turn to talk, they couldn't quite explain what my job had been. They knew it had to do with television, that I used to fly to meetings. Beyond that, they really didn't have a clue.

It's not that I hadn't told them. It's that what I did was too abstract. There was nothing you could hold in your hand for show-and-tell.

All the kids agreed on which dad had the coolest job: a guy who made screen doors. *That* was something a son or daughter could point to with pride.

I learned something from that conversation. Kids—both boys and girls—need nuts and bolts. Screwdrivers and lathes. To feel at ease in the world, they have to learn what the world is actually made of, and how it got that way.

Just as it's crucial for underprivileged kids to be shown that there are possibilities beyond their neighborhoods, it's also important for overprivileged kids to see other sides of life.

I didn't want my kids to grow up in an abstract world of deals and numbers and money that just happened. I wanted them to understand that people worked hard, at a gloriously wide range of things, and that there was dignity in all of them.

So I bought a big stretch van—my rolling locker room—and started taking my kids and their friends on what I thought of as Real World Outings. They were like school field trips, but without the onus of school. I was never "Mr. Barton." I was always Peter. I wanted the kids to be able to relax, to let off steam. If things got too rambunctious in the back of the van, I'd yell out, "Hey, what's rule number one?"

The kids would scream back, "No permanent injuries!"

And they'd settle down—a little. I loved it.

Every outing had a theme. "Grease"—where we looked closely at the realities of fast food. "Garbage"—where we followed the trail of household trash, and of recycled cars and asphalt and concrete.

One of my favorites was called "Luggage." There's a Samsonite factory in Denver; we went to it and saw the bags being made, heard the honest clank of rivets. Then we went to a retail store and asked a lot of questions: Who decided how things would be displayed? How did you figure out how many to keep in the warehouse? Who bought more luggage—men or women?

Then we drove out to the airport, having gotten permission to go "backstage" with the baggage handlers. We watched them, with their back-support belts and their elastic wristbands and their boots. Bend and jerk; bend and jerk. We saw how many suitcases they lifted, how heavy the bags were, how they just kept coming down the conveyor, relentless. . . .

Sometimes, at the end of our outings, there'd be the strangest sound in the van: silence. How rare was that? Ten or twelve kids, thinking something over.

By the time I was leading these forays, death was growing inside me. I'd outlived my father, but, by some perverse logic, that very milestone seemed to mark the beginning of my own decline. My future ended almost as soon as it started.

Still, I was thoroughly enjoying this next adventure. It was an adventure on a beautifully intimate scale. If I still had the strength and luck to accomplish anything at this stage, it wouldn't be reported in *Who's Who* or the *Wall Street Journal*. But maybe it would be scrawled here and there in a child's notebook, or etched into a young and open mind.

I could think of no better way to use the time that remained for me.

◆◆◆

YES, my working life had been quite abstract. It was about concepts. Synergies. Deals. Especially deals. I love to negotiate, and I used to think I could negotiate anything. I believed in the powers of reason and persuasion.

What does it take to be a good negotiator? There's two sides to it, I think. One side is something to be proud of; the other side is something you just have to live with. For better or worse, I had both.

The side you have to live with is an essential feistiness, a reflexive combativeness that's probably in the DNA. I don't like to lose. I can't stand feeling taken advantage of. I'd wrestle a junkyard dog for a bone I believed was rightfully mine.

But that alone doesn't make someone a good negotiator. Just a pain in the neck.

To be a good negotiator, you've got to combine that feistiness with a certain creativity. You need skill at aligning interests that, at first glance, seem opposed. You've got to structure the arrangement so that everybody wins. If I'm truly confident about anything, it's my ability to do that.

Something I've noticed, though, is that it's often the things we're good at that get us into trouble. When we're doing something we're good at, we're in a comfort zone—and we want to stay there. So we like to imagine that the thing we're good at has applications *everywhere*. We fall back on certain strategies even when we shouldn't.

So, for instance, being a confident negotiator, I felt that I could even negotiate my health. I tried to cut a deal with my own heart: I'll give you exercise, you give me time. I'll spare you cholesterol, you spare me angina.

It all seemed so logical. It all seemed so fair.

Then the cancer came along, and there was nothing logical or fair about it. It just happened. If there was a "cause," it was too complex and subtle for me to ever understand, let alone repair. Between my disease and me, there was nothing to discuss. You can't reason with a tumor.

So my illness was really a double whammy. It was grim on its own, and it also deprived me of my central tactic for dealing with life. If logic got me nowhere, if negotiating did not apply, then how was I to understand this thing that was happening to me?

That question has gnawed at me for months—no, years. It gnaws at me still. At moments I find it so frustrating that if I had the energy, I'd kick a door.

Cancer just doesn't make sense. There's a paradox here that could drive a person mad: I've spent my whole life trying to be logical, but to make peace with an illogical disease, I've got to let go of logic.

The ancients called it accepting fate. Religious people, I guess, would call it bending to the will of God. It comes down to the same thing, and it's really difficult.

I have to stop expecting explanations or justifications. I have to stop groping for some tidy piece of insight that will make all this seem fair and fitting.

I have to understand that if insight comes—the kind of mysterious, *effective* insight that trails serenity in its wake—it will not be by way of logic. Logically, I can't conclude that all is well.

Maybe peace will come by way of faith—if I can make that leap.

In the meantime, I am still a stubborn person, and my belief in reason is one of the stubbornest parts of me. And one of the things that still infuriates me about my illness is what a waste it is, what a perfect lose/lose situation.

Cancer will kill me. That much I'm resigned to. Insofar as this has been a fight, my body is the vanquished, the disease will be the victor. But it's such a hollow and inglorious triumph. Because the moment I die, the tumor starts to die as well. The cancer will have killed itself as well as me.

I think of this as an absurd and appalling bit of spite: the perfect example of a failed negotiation. An unproductive line of thought, I realize. But I happen to think it anyway. In a more reasonable world, my disease and I should really have been able to cut a deal.

18

TIME, it becomes ever clearer, is flattening out for me.

Past, present, and future no longer line up in strict, unchanging order; there's a looseness to them, a fluidity, even a playfulness that wasn't there before. Things are linked by sometimes tenuous or whimsical connections, not according to the ticking of a clock.

In part, I guess, this has to do with unwholesome changes in the chemistry of my brain, and with the abnormal rise and fall of my energy. These days it's a struggle to feel fully awake. I rest a good deal of the time but am seldom fully asleep. For hours at a stretch,

I drift along in a not-unpleasant daydream sort of state. That state has few hard edges and even fewer rules. Time can move backwards as well as forward. Or it can simply pause. I can suspend a thought, freeze a moment, hang a memory on the wall as though it were a picture—and come back to it whenever I'm ready to.

Odd, yes. But maybe inevitable. Maybe this heady blending of past and present is something that has to happen when a person considers his life *as a whole*.

It occurs to me now that we mostly live our lives facing "forward"—toward the future. Goals and consequences stretch away before us; we reach them one by one, as if we were driving down a highway. We glance into our rearview mirror now and then, but we don't truly look back until the journey's ended.

And then, of course, it all looks different. The road curved, and rose, and fell more than we had realized. The sequence wasn't half as tidy as we thought. Looking back, we see something complex but also strangely perfect. We see something *completed*.

This, I think, is a big and a quietly terrifying notion. And so people don't think about it until they're close to death.

At least I didn't. My life complete? As in finished? No, thank you. I preferred to think in terms of an ongoing progression. Choices and reactions. One thing leading to another—to the future. As long as there was a future, there had to be some arrow, some vector pointing to it.

But take away the future, and what happens to that time line?

It starts to seem like a convenient fiction. Like maybe it was never really there at all.

The past safely *behind* us? If the past is gone, where did it go?

The future suspensefully *ahead*? Ahead where? We won't know that till we get to it—and then it won't be future anymore.

I'm hardly the first person to notice that in fact there is only the present, constantly. The present moment is lived, and relived; written, and rewritten. Every previous version still inhabits it.

Besides, if the past were really behind us, why would memories have such a stubborn hold? How could a smell remembered from childhood—a musty basement, the tang of seaweed—bring a smile or a lump in the throat? Why could a song from thirty years ago still start the blood pounding in our temples and put a tingle in our loins?

Let me tell you about a day from 2000.

It was a day of pivotal events and improbable coincidences. It was the day when my future hit the wall, and past and present began piling up behind the wreckage like skidding cars in a chain collision.

In the morning of that day, I'd been to see the radiologist. This was purely routine. Since my highly successful surgery, I'd had a CT scan every three months. I always passed with flying colors. The shape of my resectioned stomach looked a little unnatural, a little weird; but other than that, my gut was clean. I'd almost stopped worrying about it.

In the late afternoon I had a visit with the doctor. Again, routine. We'd get together after every scan, quickly confirm that it showed nothing, then move on to the happier subject of my growing strength, my full recuperation.

This time it didn't go that way.

We were sitting in the consultation room, and an amazing, almost surreal, thing happened. When the doctor opened up his mouth to talk to me, his voice broke and he began to sob.

This was wildly out of keeping with the surroundings. The consultation room was designed to inspire an impersonal sort of confidence. Diplomas. Leather books. A place for expertise, not emotion.

I sat there as the doctor wept. I was flabbergasted, utterly confused. For a moment I actually imagined that we weren't going to talk about *me* at all, that the doctor was going to confess some terrible problem of his own.

Then, sniffling, he told me about the CT scan. It wasn't conclusive, he assured me. False positives did happen. But something had shown up—some shadow that did not belong there. Best case, it was a scrap of scar tissue that had tardily developed in my tampered-with belly. But it was possible that my cancer had returned. We'd have to look into it further.

I took the news quite calmly. Not because I'm brave; because I was numb and slow.

Being who I am, I tried to be rational, I considered the odds. The tests were imperfect. I was past the point when the return of cancer was a statistically probable outcome. . . . But then, why was my doctor blubbering, why did he appear so entirely crestfallen and baffled?

It's strange the way bad news sinks in. As of when I left

the consultation room, I felt matter-of-fact, almost blasé. Yes, we'd do more tests. Okay, there'd be a little worry until we proved this CT scan wrong.

By the time I reached my car, I was weak in the knees, and I knew—*knew*—that my cancer was back.

Suddenly it seemed like, in some dim way, I'd known it for a while. Hadn't felt exactly right. Was beating back dread. Was smiling through while awaiting some grim confirmation.

The confirmation, in a crazy way, was almost a relief. I now knew where I stood.

◆ ◆ ◆

I'VE SAID THIS WAS A DAY of odd coincidences, a day when many different layers of my life were squeezed onto a wafer of the present.

I didn't go home after my visit with the doctor. It so happened that the Rolling Stones were playing Denver that night. I'd been looking forward to the concert for weeks, and a little thing like cancer wasn't going to make me miss it.

I went downtown to meet Laura and some friends for dinner. I had already decided that, for the moment, I would keep my day a secret. I didn't want to ruin the evening for everyone else. Especially since the news I'd gotten had absolutely not ruined it for me.

Just the opposite, in fact. I was jazzed. I felt intensely alive. Every pore was open; every sensation was heightened. The worst was happening, and I was staring it down. I was scared but I was happy.

At the restaurant, I said my hellos and then stared at my wife.

Married couples, however much in love they are, tend to fall into habitual ways of seeing each other. Sometimes it takes a shock to make perception new again. In that moment, I didn't see Laura as my companion of the past fifteen years and the mother of my children. I saw her as the woman I wanted to marry *now*. She looked beautiful. She laughed with everyone, put everyone at ease. She had the most natural kind of confidence, a poise that was totally informal.

I hugged her. In the midst of the hug, some very hard thoughts flowed through me. What would my death be like for her?

She'd think of the kids first, of course, but still. . . . How would she deal with seeing me weaken and fade? How would she bear up in the face of my frustrations and crankiness? How would she face the burdens of being a young widow with three children?

I blinked back the tears that hadn't come when I was with the doctor, hid the sniffles behind a pretended sneeze, and sat down to have dinner with our friends.

We were a motley crew—some mountain-biking buddies, a pro-boxing promoter, and a couple of Olympic fighters. We talked sports and music and put away prodigious amounts of food.

I ate like I hadn't eaten in decades. I ate like I was going to the chair. I didn't worry about cholesterol. I didn't worry about my compromised stomach. Friends who knew my usually abstemious habits looked at me sideways. I flashed them a glance that said, *What? Haven't you ever seen a person wolf down a giant cheeseburger, two orders of fries, and a pitcher of beer before?*

We headed to the concert.

I'm not sure I'd ever really believed that there would be a "last" Rolling Stones concert. But now here it was—if not for the band, then almost certainly for me. It dawned on me that a totally weird series of events was beginning. From now on, I'd start doing the *last* this and the *last* that.

What a wild notion.

Life is finite. We all know that, and we conveniently forget about it almost every hour of almost every day. But now the fact was in my face, a granite monolith across my field of vision. With the future sealed off, past and present bounced off of it and swirled.

The process started almost before we were inside the gates. I ran into my old friend John Sykes, the guy who runs VH-1. We laughed about another Stones concert we'd both attended—the 1994 tour opener at Shea Stadium.

I'd been running Liberty then. I was at the height of my career, and also the height of my chutzpah. I'd had a media pass and a great seat way up front. But that hadn't been good enough for me. I was still the kid who had to push the limits, to find a

208 • NOT FADE AWAY

way past every velvet rope. I kept flashing my pass, talking my way around security guards, getting deeper and deeper into the heart of the event—until I was right up on the stage! I strolled around among the Rolling Stones' guitars and amps. Then I casually sat down next to Eric Clapton. We got to chatting. I bet him a beer he didn't have the nerve to break in and play a solo. He grabbed a spare guitar and played an epic forty-five-minute riff. His hand was still hot when I handed him the brew.

Can I explain the crazy richness of that experience? I was up there because I was supposedly a media business big shot, but in my heart I was a groupie, a total wide-eyed fan. In the same instant, I was a grown-up wheeler-dealer and a goofy teenager once again—the same kid who'd gotten goose bumps when he'd seen the Hoffner bass his father gave him.

Past and present captured in a heartbeat. My whole life vibrant and precious before my eyes.

Now it was 2000. I was a civilian again, sitting not with the VIPs but in the throbbing middle of a vast communal audience— an audience like the huge, electric gatherings of the sixties—another layer of experience that was with me always. I was a sick man, but, in the alternate present of memory, still a manic, hopeful youth. My day had been a dirge, but now I was up for rock 'n' roll.

The music started. "Brown Sugar." It was pulsing. It was loud. It was the same as it had ever been. Which is to say, not the greatest music ever written, not performed by the most fabulous musicians, but totally compelling, utterly true to what it was. It was rough; it was rude. It was the soundtrack of my life, made of yearning and rebellion. It was the screaming garage band raised to the sublime.

And if there was a tinge of irony in how Mick Jagger performed these days—why not? The man was middle-aged, for God's sake! Maybe he too was seeing his life as a giddy mix of past and present. Maybe, like me, he was taking sustenance from the thought of how much *then* survived into the *now*, how remarkably durable an old self is.

Durable enough, maybe, to survive even death.

The place rocked on. The audience became a happy mob, swaying together, stomping. Remembering how good it felt to feel that good. Savoring our luck in having had those songs, those ill-behaved and sacred anthems of our youth.

The concert ended. The band left the stage. The roars and screams of thousands brought them back for an encore. An old song; one of the greatest. Out of tune, off the beat—and perfect!—a great huddle of humanity sang along.

> *Love is love and not fade away.*
> *Love is love and not fade away.*
> *Love is love and not fade away.*

I joined in, of course. I always joined in. I brought forth a joyous sound from deep down in my damaged belly. I sang it out till I was hoarse and weeping.

19

AND NOW MY STORY is almost over.

Its two strands—the story of my life, the story of my illness—have nearly come together.

I've wanted to believe, I guess, that they'd keep running parallel forever, stretching like a pair of tracks toward a wide horizon that could never be reached. But that isn't how it works in life.

In life, all story lines eventually converge. The adventure that began with my birth in 1951 will end at the exact moment and in the same manner as the drama that started on Pearl Harbor Day of 1998.

Death is the completion. Death is where the horizon finally stops receding. Not a separate thing from life, but life's last resolving chord.

That chord is coming close. I can almost hear it.

In these pages, I have deliberately avoided saying very much about the physical details of my cancer. Such details are highly unpleasant, even gruesome, and not especially edifying. Lately, though, the physical fact of my illness has become so striking, so *present*, that I can't sweep it aside any longer.

These days I can see my tumor. I've become so thin, and the tumor has grown so robust, that its outline is clearly visible beneath my skin. It has a crescent-shaped edge, like some appalling rind. It presses against the incisions from my various procedures. At moments it threatens to stretch open the sutures.

I don't want to be morbid, but I find a horrid fascination in the sheer bulk of my illness.

People tend to think of disease as microscopic and abstract. My cancer is no longer anything like that. My cancer has become a *thing*, material and obvious. It has weight and volume. Like every object, it has to *be* somewhere, and as it claims more space it is evicting me from my own body. My disease, literally, is taking my place.

The process, by this point, is largely mechanical. It involves friction, and pressure, and squeezing. But the pain, for the most part, is manageable these days. The narcotics keep me in a zone that I think of as a humming discomfort. I don't feel right, but I don't feel terrible.

Now and then, a spike of real agony breaks through. The aftermath of these spikes is far worse than the pain itself. I perceive it less as pain than as loss of balance, loss of orientation—loss of connection with myself. In the wake of every breakthrough episode, I feel dizzy and a little panicked. My heart races, I break into a clammy sweat. I feel like I might die.

But enough. The bad stuff can't go on much longer. Besides, these are merely physical complaints, and the good news—the *real* news—is that my long quest to move beyond the physical has nearly been accomplished. My poor old body is only a detail these days. My flesh has less and less to do with who I am.

I've been letting go, and this . . . yes, I'll call it a surrender . . . this surrender has been accompanied by something strange and wonderful. I'm not sure I can adequately describe it. But let me look for words that will at least come close.

A kind of singing quiet has been settling over me.

It arrived unbidden. It took me by surprise. I've had neither strength nor inclination to fight it off or question it.

Maybe this quiet is nothing more or less than what some people mean by acceptance. Or peace. Or grace. But there's a richness to it, a texture, that I did not expect.

It isn't passive; only still. It's close to death yet full of life.

For me, this quiet is another form of music. It's music without motion, just a harmony frozen in time.

I wish I could explain how I've finally arrived at this

amazing calm. Truthfully, though, I suspect that I did not *achieve* this quiet, or even find it. It found me when the time was right.

I think over the years of my illness—no, over my entire life—and I consider my flailing efforts to find serenity. I chased it with logic, but at the same time used logic to fend it off. I sought it with yearning, with private rituals that were my own eccentric way of praying, of moving closer to the spiritual.

Now I feel that these exercises, while necessary, were probably beside the point. Peace keeps its own schedule. You can't hurry it. And when it comes, it's a gift freely given, more than something earned.

My hunch is that it comes to saints and sinners equally. It's not about justice, and it doesn't mean that life is fair. Just inevitable.

A big part of the calm that has settled over me is the happy conviction that my wife and children will be okay. I don't know if this belief is a cause or an effect of my serenity, and it really doesn't matter. What matters is that, after my wrenching sorrow at leaving Laura and the kids, after my aching guilt about what my sickness has put them through, I have come to feel a proud confidence that they will emerge from this with their spirits intact and a great deal of wonderful life ahead of them.

I'm sorry for the worry I've caused, and for the grieving that is still ahead. But I also know that grief will subside, that at some point memories will bring thoughtful smiles along with the tears.

I hope and trust that my family will continue to feel love for me. I believe that love can reach past loss and make their lives richer. Absent, I can still be part of who they are. Grieving is part of loving. That's just how it is.

As for the rest . . . I've poured myself into my life. I haven't held back. And I've pretty well used myself up.

This calm I feel now—in some ways it's a more durable case of the contented exhaustion I have felt after skiing for ten hours, or playing music through the night, or working round the clock at something that seemed terribly important at the time. It's a calm that comes from knowing that I've held nothing back.

I've worked hard at my life. I'm proud of that. None of it came easily, and sometimes I pursued it with more insistence than grace. But that's who I have always been, and I'm proud of that as well.

If I had pushed a little less, relaxed a little more, I might have led a longer life—who knows? But I could not have had a life that suited me better, a life that was more my own. I'm very grateful.

There's just one final thing I want to say. Probably it's how everybody wants to be remembered. But that's okay. I've said from the start that I make no claim of being special; I'm just one more person dying, revisiting his life. I think my father would have said the same thing, in the same words, if he'd had the time.

It's simply this: I really tried. I did my best.

EPILOGUE

ON AUGUST 29, 2002, Peter, along with his wife and three children, flew to New York to attend the annual MTV Video Music Awards, held at Radio City Music Hall.

Peter was quite weak by then. The tumor that was still expanding in his abdomen had encased his liver and made it clog with bile; his skin and eyes were turning a morbid yellow-orange. But he badly wanted to make this trip. He'd talked about it for weeks. The kids were excited. Kate and Jeff had attended the awards in previous years and thought of the evening as a second Christmas. But the youngest child, Chris, had never gone. This was a last great opportunity to etch a family memory.

At Radio City, Peter was offered a wheelchair to take him to his seat. He declined, and walked the red carpet into the vast auditorium, steadying himself with a bony hand on the armrests of each row. During a commercial break in the broadcast, the MTV host, Carson Daly, made a short speech, thanking Peter for believing in MTV from the beginning, and for his role in helping to create the cable television industry that made all this possible. Six thousand people stood and applauded.

The next day, Peter took his family on a carriage ride through Central Park. A photograph was taken. Framed by the awning of the hansom cab, Peter, behind big sunglasses, surrounded by his family, is smiling broadly, his arms thrown open in a wide, encompassing embrace. Nine days later he was dead.

The steep decline began almost the moment he returned to Denver—and I have to believe that Peter knew it would. This, remember, was a man who could negotiate almost anything, and I think he cut a final deal with life. If life would give him one more perfect family trip, he would finally stop struggling, he would gratefully let go.

After a last sunset watched with a small group of friends, Peter took to his bed. He lay there motionless, and, over the next week, as the toxins built up in his blood, his awareness became sporadic, his voice gravelly and soft. In one of his last brief conversations, he told Laura that he was on a beautiful ship. She asked him where the ship was going. He smiled faintly, coyly, and said it was a secret.

At length he lost the ability to speak, then even the power to acknowledge others speaking. His breath grew ever shallower. Peter, who had drunk so deeply of life, now subsisted on mere hurried sips of air.

He slipped into a light and timeless sleep—a state in which his thoughts could only be guessed, and the guesses would reveal far more about the hopes and fears of the observer than about Peter himself. What was happening to him had at last become unknowable.

On Sunday, September 8, 2002, at around nine-thirty in the morning, Peter Barton died.

As was his wish, he passed away at home, connected to no monitors or life-support equipment. His wife and daughter were at his bedside; his sons were rattling around the house, making the noise that Peter loved to hear. Laura brought them in to see their father in repose. He was five months and two days past his fifty-first birthday.

In keeping with a plan that he and Laura had tearfully, joyfully arrived at, the body he'd left behind was dressed in his pink and white striped birthing shirt to be cremated. A week later, in a small family ceremony, his ashes were buried in a cemetery meadow high up in the Rocky Mountains.

* * *

FROM ALMOST OUR FIRST CONVERSATION, Peter had insisted that there was nothing special in the fact of his dying, that his mortality mattered neither more nor less than that of the billions of people who had passed away before. Dying was sad, but it happened to everyone, and in precisely equal measure. Death, he felt, came in one size only.

The same cannot be said of lives. There are smaller lives and larger lives, and the surest gauge of the scale of a life is how many other lives it touches. By this standard, Peter had lived big.

His passing was major news in Denver, where it was reported not just in obituary notices but in long feature articles in both the *Denver Post* and the *Rocky Mountain News*. The *New York Times* and the *Los Angeles Times* saluted Peter as a media pioneer.

This official recognition was impressive . . . and yet it seemed oddly impersonal, beside the point. Peter would have been more pleased, I think, to see the hundreds of friends who rallied around his family. Kids he'd coached, or taken along on his Real World Outings. Colleagues he'd advised and schemed with. Neighbors whose dogs had gotten muddy alongside Peter's dogs. People he'd skied with, or biked with, or with whom he'd sat around the piano and jammed and wailed.

More than fifteen hundred of these friends and colleagues and acquaintances turned out for Peter's memorial—an event intended not for mourning but for celebration. There was a gospel choir, and a children's choir in which Kate sang. There was food and wine. There was a stitched-together video of Peter's life, accompanied—of course!—by a rock 'n' roll soundtrack. And there were speeches.

In keeping with the spirit of the evening, the speakers passed lightly over the subject of Peter sick and dying, still seeking meaning in the face of pain and honest doubt. Instead, they spoke of Peter in his glory. Peter, who believed that nothing was impossible. Peter, who could step into a situation, overwhelmed but never daunted, and master it. Peter, who skied too fast, drove too fast, worked too hard, and made it all look easy.

I listened to the eulogies and was reminded how extraordinarily varied and how relentlessly active Peter's life had been. But I realized something else as well. For all their insight and affection, none of the speakers quite conjured up the Peter I had known, the man who had become my friend in the last months of his life.

Other friends had run with Peter; Peter and I sat still together. Other friends, looking to the future, had made big plans with him, had pieced together empires; with Peter and me, it was usually just the two of us, looking backward, talking quietly, trying to decide what was of value and what was not.

I mourned the sides of Peter I had not had time to know; I'd missed a lot of what had made him so remarkable. At the same time, I was touched and proud to realize how rare and privileged my own glimpse of him had been. I understood that I needed to say a more personal good-bye.

◆◆◆

THE NEXT MORNING, I drove west from Denver, heading for the mountains.

It was the eighteenth of September. The aspens were just turning, painting slashes of yellow onto hillsides blanketed in the heavy green of spruce and pine. Before dawn, the season's first snow had fallen. Above nine thousand feet, it still bearded the trees and softened the contours of granite faces.

Driving, my thoughts and feelings were a muddle; I let them stay that way. I wondered about the mystery of Peter's final hours; in my fashion, I prayed that he had clung to his resolve to cross over with joy, to see death as an adventure. I mulled over the odd custom of visiting a grave site. What of Peter had actually been buried? Only ashes. His soul—if one believed that it existed—existed everywhere. Why, then, did a visit to the grave seem so important, necessary?

It was snowing again as I crossed the Divide. Clouds closed in, then parted, then closed in once more; warm sun made each new flurry gleam silver. I continued toward Vail Pass—the part of the Rockies that Peter loved above all others. He used to say that when he was up here, skiing or hiking, he felt that he was poised between earth and heaven.

On the Interstate, and then on a rutted, unpaved road that snaked away into wilderness, I climbed up to eleven thousand feet.

Peter's grave is in a tiny cemetery embedded in a forest. Behind a simple iron gate, a small meadow leads on toward a row of spruces. A break in the trees reveals a second clearing. Here, I'd been told, was where I would find my friend's resting place. There was no stone yet, no marker; I would recognize the grave only by the freshly turned earth.

But the earth itself had now been buried under a foot or more of snow. I knew I was close to Peter's grave; whether I actually reached it I have no idea. This was a humbling irony I know Peter would have savored; standing there knee-deep, I could almost hear him chuckling over it: We humans try so hard to reach our goals, to do the things our hearts tell us need doing, and even as we're doing them we don't know if we're succeeding.

But no matter. I was standing in the meadow that Peter had chosen as his final earthly home, and I felt his presence very clearly. I saw him once again at the piano, beating back mortality with big loud chords. I heard him protesting that he wasn't spiritual, wasn't introspective, then making a liar of himself in every conversation. I saw him weep when he talked about how much he would miss his family.

Then I, in turn, was surprised by tears. I felt them as hot rivulets against the cold of falling snow. I heard my own small voice break into the stupendous silence of the forest. "Peter, it's been great," I said. "I wish I knew you longer."

I turned away and headed down the mountain.

ACKNOWLEDGMENTS

WRITING IS A REMARKABLY LONELY and solitary pursuit—and I came to love that about it. I loved the time when there was nothing in the world other than me, a word processor, and a dog or two underfoot. In the loneliness I found a quiet spot where I could think, reflect, and discover what this story was truly meant to say.

Yet certain people were with me even during those solitary hours. Family has always been the most important part of my life, and I want to thank the people who made me what I am: my Mom and short-lived Dad, and my two wonderful brothers, John and Tom. My dear friend David Koff and my best friend Laura Barton inspired me by their own high standards and their belief that this book could be of value. Larry Shames, partner and friend, proved to be a marvelously accomplished and insightful storyteller.

This project also brought me into contact with Stephen White, a very special man and come-lately soul-mate. A best-selling fiction writer, Stephen is also a former chef, clinical psychologist, and pain-management specialist. He is one of the most vital intellects and generous men I have ever met.

Finally, for his amazing spirit and the example of his courage, my gratitude goes out to Mac Elliman, a young man who for so many years has inspired us all to make the most of each opportunity to smile. —*P.B.*

This book, from its conception, has had the great good fortune to be met not only with understanding but with passion. I would like to thank everyone at Rodale for a level of commitment that has become a rare luxury in contemporary publishing. In particular, my gratitude is owed to Marc Jaffe, for his deeply personal interest; to Amy Rhodes, for her wholehearted and imaginative support; to Chris Potash, for his tireless work with the manuscript; and, most of all, to Stephanie Tade, whose boundless caring and enthusiasm have made her the sort of champion that every author dreams of having.

I'd like to thank my agent, Stuart Krichevsky, for believing in this story and in my ability to set it down. I am grateful to Cathie Wlaschin, Peter's long-time assistant, for her careful gathering of his archives. My thanks, as well, to the many friends of Peter's who shared impressions and reminiscences with me. I hope I've done some measure of justice to the man they all remembered with such wonder and such love. —*L.S.*